'This is a book that has been needed for some time and te Brian is the perfect person to have written it. Pregnancy and parenting following the losses and lack of control brought about by infertility, and many rounds of assisted conception procedures, *is* different. Kate combines her own personal experience with quotes from experts and stories from IVF recipients – and their children – with common sense, humour and a style that is knowledgeable, warm and very accessible. I recommend this book to parents of all precious babies, including those conceived with the help of a donor – you will find much here to reassure you.'
Olivia Montuschi, co-founder of Donor Conception Network and mother to two donor-conceived adults

'This book is full of sensible advice for couples who conceive after struggling with infertility. Kate Brian uses real-life cases histories to illustrate the issues that arise during pregnancy, childbirth and when parenting children who result from fertility treatment. Interspersed with sensible and relevant advice from recognised experts in the field, *Precious Babies* is both readable and informative. It explores areas that many of us who work with infertile couples either take for granted or assume will be dealt with later in the process of pregnancy management. Although there is wisdom in the quotation from the book "Just because I'd had problems getting pregnant, it didn't mean that I had to have problems being pregnant", pregnancies arising from fertility treatment are doubly precious and the common sense approach, backed up with evidence, that Kate Brian uses in her book will be a boon to all couples who achieve a pregnancy after infertility.'
Professor Bill Ledger, University of New South Wales

'Kate Brian has addressed an enormously important but overlooked aspect of infertility in exploring the impact that continues even after successful treatment results in a pregnancy and parenthood. With her unique ability to blend personal stories, expert views and medical and scientific information she provides answers to the many questions that arise as soon as a pregnancy is confirmed. Prompted by her own experience she gets to the heart of what women want to know about the practicalities of having a baby and astutely confronts the concerns so widely experienced but rarely articulated. With insight and sensitivity, *Precious Babies* explains why it is different having a baby after fertility treatment and explores the mixed emotions of great joy but also anxiety and psychological complexities in parenting these children. What makes it a real treasure is that the book exudes reassurance that you are not alone and builds confidence with a strong, positive voice. *Precious Babies* is not only an invaluable resource for women, their partners, families and friends but essential reading for all professionals involved with caring for them, from those providing infertility services, midwives and obstetricians through to the wider community.'

Jane Denton, director, The Multiple Births Foundation

PRECIOUS BABIES

Pregnancy, Birth and
Parenting after Infertility

KATE BRIAN

piatkus

PIATKUS

First published in Great Britain in 2011 by Piatkus

A CIP catalogue record for this book
is available from the British Library.

ISBN 978-0-7499-5401-7

Typeset in ITC Esprit by Palimpsest Book Production Limited,
Falkirk, Stirlingshire
Printed and bound in Great Britain by Clays Ltd, St Ives plc

Papers used by Piatkus are from well-managed forests
and other responsible sources.

MIX
Paper from
responsible sources
FSC
www.fsc.org FSC® C104740

Piatkus
An imprint of
Little, Brown Book Group
100 Victoria Embankment
London EC4Y 0DY

An Hachette UK Company
www.hachette.co.uk

www.piatkus.co.uk

To Alfie and Flora, my very precious babies

Kate Brian specialises in issues surrounding fertility, and is the author of *The Complete Guide to Female Fertility* and *The Complete Guide to IVF*. She was awarded for her work for Infertility Network UK, and has been closely involved with the charity for many years. Kate works as a freelance writer and editor, and regularly appears on TV and radio as an expert on fertility. She has two children who were born after IVF treatment.

Contents

3. Miscarriage   59

Acknowledgements

Thank you to all those who gave up their time to talk to me when I was researching this book. I am so grateful to you for offering to share your experiences in order to help others, and for your honesty. It was wonderful to hear the stories of so many precious babies!

I would also like to thank the professionals who agreed to give their expert advice: special thanks to Tarek El-Toukhy of Guy's and St Thomas' Hospital, Professor Bill Ledger of the University of New South Wales, Jane Denton of The Multiple Births Foundation, Olivia Montuschi of the Donor Conception Network, Professor James Walker of the Royal College of Obstetricians and Gynaecologists, Ruth Bender-Atik of The Miscarriage Association, Professor Susan Golombok of the Centre for Family Research at the University of Cambridge, Mollie Graneek of BICA, Dr Ellie Lee of the Centre for Parenting Culture Studies at the University of Kent, Dr Karin Hammarberg of the University of Melbourne, Dr Geetha Venkat of the Harley Street Fertility Clinic, Caroline Rice of TAMBA, Manjit Randhawa of St Thomas' Hospital, Lindsey Harris of mothers35plus. co.uk, Gerad Kite and Dr Bernice Sorensen.

I owe a huge thank you to Clare Lewis-Jones MBE, Chief Executive of ACeBabes and Infertility Network UK, for being such a great source of support and inspiration, and to all the wonderful staff I worked with at the charity – Alison Onash, Claire Ogilvie, Diane Arnold, Fiona O'Donnell, Gwenda Burns, Helene Torr, Sharon Davidson, Sheena Young, Susan Seenan and Tracey Sainsbury.

I am very grateful to Anne Lawrence at Piatkus who championed this idea from the outset and has been a truly fabulous editor. My thanks to everyone else at Piatkus who has been involved with the book, especially Jillian Stewart, and thanks to Jan Cutler. I would also like to thank Diana Tyler, my agent at MBA, who has stuck with me throughout.

Finally, I owe a huge debt of gratitude to all my friends and family who have endured yet another book; particularly Daphne McCord, Anna McCord and Christine Oldfield. As ever, my love and greatest thanks are saved for Max, Alfie and Flora.

Foreword

When Kate told me she was writing *Precious Babies* my immediate reaction was that this was a much needed and overdue book and therefore I welcome it wholeheartedly. It takes you from that wonderful moment when you find out you are pregnant, to what can sadly go wrong and how to look after yourself during pregnancy, through to giving birth and parenting after infertility. It is a book that answers many of the questions that perhaps we are too nervous to ask for fear of appearing neurotic or daft!

In my work as Chief Executive of Infertility Network UK, the national patient organisation for those affected by difficulties in conceiving, I hear from and speak to those affected every day – including those who have had successful treatment. As this book makes clear, the emotional impact of infertility is enormous and is often compared to bereavement by counsellors, psychologists and psychotherapists. That huge emotional impact doesn't just go away once you find out you are pregnant. As Kate says, most people have been trying for a number of years and have experienced so much failure in their efforts to have a family that it's not surprising that they are almost expecting it to go wrong again. It can sometimes be difficult to know exactly how to play it. Should you expect failure so that if something does go wrong somehow it won't hit you so hard? Or should you think positively so that those positive 'vibes' will somehow stop something going wrong? But then, if it does go wrong, will you then feel even worse?

That is most certainly how I felt as I was going through treatment – totally confused on how best to deal with possible failure or success. And for many this can go on for several years, which takes a huge emotional toll. For those reasons, amongst others, my charity also includes ACeBabes as part of our network of support. People were contacting us saying that whilst they were delighted they were pregnant, they still had worries and concerns yet could not go back to the support group they used to go to, as it might upset those who were still trying. We recognised the fact that people who conceive or adopt following infertility still need to know that there is support out there from people who understand why they may be feeling frightened or alone. They truly benefit from speaking to others on our forums and from meeting up with other families, achieved after struggling to conceive.

Over the course of nine years of trying for a child, investigations, tubal surgery and finally three attempts at IVF, I imagined what it would be like to finally have a family. The treatment didn't work and I then pursued adoption – successfully – and adopted my two children, James and Holly. I always say, and truly believe, that we were meant to go through those years of treatment so that we were there for our children when they needed us – it was fate! But now all of a sudden we had what we'd been trying to achieve for such a long time and I really did try to be a super-parent. I felt I couldn't complain about how tired I was, or what a difficult day I'd had and worried about whether I'd handled a situation like the perfect mother or not. But my husband isn't Superman and I am certainly not Wonder Woman, though we tried to be. My children are grown up now but even so, I still found the book reassuring in terms of how we coped when we had our family.

There is absolutely no doubt that infertility and its treatment puts you on an emotional rollercoaster and sometimes you wonder if you will ever get off it. For this reason, solid practical information and emotional support is vital, and this book provides just that. Kate has been there herself, thus treats the subject and those affected sympathetically and with understanding. Every aspect is covered in a practical way and is backed up with advice from experts in the field. The personal stories are equally important and helpful – again, illustrating that you are not alone in how you may be feeling, but also providing information and advice so that you feel empowered to move forward.

I send you my congratulations if you have just found out you are pregnant. I am so pleased you found this book, as I know you will benefit from it, not just now but over the coming years as your family gets older, and perhaps grows, and you pick it up from time to time.

Clare Lewis-Jones MBE
Chief Executive
Infertility Network UK, ACeBabes and More To Life

Introduction

Ever since I discovered I was finally pregnant after many years trying to conceive, I've been aware of the need for this book. When we were having fertility treatment, I had imagined that the impact of our fertility problems would simply disappear from our lives if we ever achieved that much longed-for pregnancy. In fact, the grey veil that had overshadowed everything lifted very quickly, but pregnancy hadn't miraculously erased the past and I didn't feel just the same as any other pregnant woman.

I had dreamt of being pregnant for so long, envisaging a blissfully happy time, but in fact my joy was submerged in anxiety. I kept comparing myself with other women I knew who were also expecting and wondering why I didn't have the relaxed attitude that they all seemed to adopt. Unlike them, I didn't dare to feel certain that I was going to have a baby at the end of my pregnancy and I was forever worried about tempting fate if I bought things for the baby or started to get a room ready. Of course, all pregnant women worry, but I was aware that my anxiety was on another scale altogether and that some of my concerns verged on the ridiculous. I read pregnancy books convinced that I had every complication under the sun and felt that my body, which had failed to get pregnant for so long, was bound to be pretty useless at carrying a baby too. I had got so used to being disappointed that I didn't feel able to enjoy pregnancy properly, despite the fact that it was all I had wanted for so long.

It wasn't until I started talking to other people who hadn't found it easy to get pregnant that I realised my reaction wasn't unusual. Infertility can make you lose confidence and self-belief and it takes time to rebuild those things once you are pregnant. Even after the birth of your baby, the past can continue to have an impact. Once my son was born I was full of joy and delight but, like many others who had taken time to conceive, I had ridiculously high expectations, trying to be a perfect parent at all times. Feeling tired or fed up simply wasn't permissable. It wasn't so much that I wouldn't admit to any negative feelings but more that I wouldn't allow any such thoughts to even enter my head. I still found it hard to believe that we really had a baby and that he was there to stay, and I felt I had to relish every nappy change and nighttime wakening.

In this book, I've tried to address some of the issues that arise for those of us who have waited a long time for our babies, and to give some practical suggestions about how to help. There's advice on trying for another child, on multiple births and donor-conceived families, on miscarriage and on having an only child. I've included a chapter on postnatal depression too, which is just as common among women who've experienced infertility in the past but can come as far more of a shock to a mother who feels pressure to be constantly filled with joy once she has a baby.

The book includes stories from parents throughout, who give honest and open accounts of their own very different experiences of pregnancy, birth and parenting after infertility. Of course, there's lots of information about the early days, but I think it's important to recognise the ways in which the sometimes subtle differences of being a parent to a long-awaited child can continue for many years. I've looked at how people tell their children about their conception, and at some of the common threads that run through our experiences as parents, from concerns about being overprotective to the demands that we put on ourselves as we try to be perfect parents. I've tried to balance the emotional aspects of this with practical tips and advice from leading experts in the field as well as other parents to ensure that anyone who has waited for their child will find something that will help them in these pages.

It may have taken me 15 years to finally get around to writing this book and finding a sympathetic publisher, but my conviction that the book is needed hasn't faded at all since those early weeks of my first pregnancy. For most parents who have taken time to get pregnant, the pain of infertility disappears fairly quickly, but when you emerge from the other side you are inevitably a different person because of what you have been through, and a different type of parent too. Once the initial anxieties, concerns and desire for perfection have passed, these differences can be positive rather than negative but we don't always see that ourselves.

My aim in writing this book is to help others who are experiencing that mix of excitement and anxiety, joy and disbelief, and who are feeling that they aren't quite the same as other parents despite appearances. I hope this book will answer some of your questions and provide useful information, but more than anything I hope it will help you realise that you are not alone and that others experience similar feelings and emotions. I feel it is important not to let our past experiences become a burden, or to continue to see them in a negative light, but instead to try to focus on some of the good things that have been left in the wake. Our children are very wanted and loved, and we know the value of what we have. We don't take our families for granted, and we are able to appreciate the wonderful gift we have been given in our truly precious babies.

CHAPTER 1

The Long-awaited Positive Result

Congratulations! When you've spent some time trying to get pregnant, finally achieving a positive pregnancy-test result is a moment you will have dreamt of. Whether you have been through years of tests and treatment or have just been worried about your fertility for a while, there have probably been times when you wondered whether you would ever get a positive test result. Reaching your goal can feel like the end of a long and exhausting odyssey, with many trials and traumas along the way.

For those of us who didn't get pregnant easily, a positive test result can bring an overwhelming mix of emotions as our minds race through feelings of disbelief, amazement, joy and elation. You may have always imagined that if you ever got to this point, the years of pain that had gone before would simply disappear and you would immediately become exactly the same as any other newly pregnant woman. In purely physical terms, it is absolutely true that the way your baby was conceived need not make any difference once the tiny embryo has implanted itself into the walls of the womb and is starting to grow; however, you may be worlds apart from other expectant parents emotionally. For you, this moment is the peak of many years of expectation and anticipation, the result of a huge emotional, and often financial, investment and this will inevitably alter your perspective. The fallout may continue to follow you not just through the pregnancy and birth but is also likely to have some impact on your life for years to come, although it may turn into a positive force in the future.

Getting the result

Discovering you are finally pregnant is a life experience that will be etched on your mind forever. My positive result came after four years of trying to conceive, which is not such a long time in the scheme of things, although it certainly hadn't felt that way at the time. We'd been through the emotional upheaval of an unsuccessful IVF cycle, followed by an unsuccessful frozen embryo transfer, so I was steeling myself for the inevitable when the time came to do the test. Like most women who've had fertility problems, I'd taken dozens of pregnancy tests over the years, every one of them negative – I'd waited for non-existent lines to appear in the windows of little plastic kits, and imagined phantom pregnancy symptoms. Over time, the one thing I'd grown accustomed to was living with the disappointment of not being pregnant, and the one thing I had no idea how to handle was a positive pregnancy-test result.

I'd got up early on the great day of testing, unable to sleep, wanting to get it over and done with. I watched as one dark blue line appeared in the little window of the plastic test kit, and then a second, equally dark blue, line. I was so braced for disappointment that initially I didn't even register that this was what I'd spent so long waiting for. All my usual coping-with-disappointment thoughts began to spring into my mind, and then it suddenly struck me that I'd never seen two blue lines before, and that this meant the result was positive.

I'd always thought I'd jump into the air screaming and shouting with joy if a test ever came up positive. Instead, I just immediately assumed that there was something wrong with the testing kit. I've since discovered that I wasn't alone in having this kind of reaction. Women I've interviewed have worked their way through dozens of pregnancy testing kits when they've had a positive result after experiencing fertility problems, convinced that every kit must be faulty because they've got recurrent positive results. By this stage you are so used to things going wrong that you have all your strategies in place for dealing with yet more of the same, and a positive result is uncharted territory.

'The treatment had gone really well, but I didn't dare to think, even to myself, that it might have worked. We did a home test but I couldn't bear to look at the result and I made my partner check it. When he said I was pregnant, we couldn't believe it. I did a test almost every day until

I had my first scan, because I kept thinking they would start showing up negative. Even that didn't make me feel confident though. I think we were in a state of shock.'

Harriet

Could a positive result after a home test be wrong?

Although many of us find it quite hard to believe that our first ever positive test could be correct, today's home pregnancy tests are extremely accurate as long as you have followed the instructions properly. They work by checking for the pregnancy hormone HCG (human chorionic gonadotropin), which your body will start to produce as soon as you are pregnant. It is very rare to get a false positive result from a home pregnancy test, unless you have been taking HCG as part of your treatment. If you are taking HCG, the fertility clinic should have made this quite clear to you, and will have explained that it would affect a home pregnancy test.

A false negative result is sometimes a possibility, however, especially if you have been unable to resist testing earlier than you should have done. The test instructions may advise that it is best to do it first thing in the morning or to avoid drinking too much liquid beforehand, and it is important to follow these directions if you want to be sure of a clear result.

The expert view

Tarek El-Toukhy, consultant in reproductive medicine, Guy's and St Thomas' Hospital

'We recommend that the earliest a home pregnancy test should be done is 15–16 days after egg collection with IVF or ICSI. The reference point should be egg collection rather than embryo transfer, because patients may not all have embryo transfer at the same stage; for example, if they have blastocyst transfer, this will be later. We don't recommend doing a test earlier than this because you could get a false negative by doing that and you could end up being unnecessarily disappointed. You can't get a false positive by testing early. If the hormone levels are high enough to register, then you would be pregnant.

'Generally, home pregnancy tests are very reliable now. If a patient is pregnant, there can sometimes be a false negative result but that happens in less than 5 per cent of cases. If patients do a first test which is negative and their period doesn't start, we recommend that they should repeat the test again in 48 hours.

'It is not usually possible to get a false positive result. This would only happen if the clinic had suggested supporting the luteal phase of the cycle with HCG injections instead of progesterone. In that case it would actually be an induced positive result and not a false positive result. It would only show a faint line and the clinic should have told the patient that a urine test would not be reliable because of the HCG injections anyway.

continued

> The drugs used in a normal IVF cycle won't affect the outcome of a pregnancy test. HCG injections during the luteal phases are the only drugs that can do this by inducing a false positive.'

Pregnancy blood tests

Some fertility clinics like you to have a blood test as well as testing at home, but this isn't always necessary, as urine tests are so accurate. The advantage of a blood test is that it can give a good indication of the level of hormones in your blood; if the levels are high, this may suggest a multiple pregnancy, whereas a lower level may suggest that the pregnancy is not going to be viable or that it could be ectopic. If there are any concerns about your pregnancy, the medical team will usually ask you to return for a series of blood tests to see whether the hormone levels are rising normally, as this would indicate that everything is progressing well. You can always ask for a pregnancy blood test if you'd like the extra reassurance, but you may be expected to pay for this yourself, as it tends to be seen as a luxury rather than a necessity. If you've had a previous ectopic pregnancy, however, your doctor may suggest carrying out a series of pregnancy blood tests to rule out any risk of another ectopic.

I was scheduled to have a blood test later on the day of my first positive home test. I spent the day on tenterhooks waiting for the clinic to ring with the result, unable to believe that the home test could possibly be correct. Even when the nurse had told me that the blood test confirmed that I was pregnant, I was still plagued with irrational doubts about the hospital mixing up my blood test with someone else's results. At least having an official confirmation did stop me buying half a dozen more home pregnancy-test kits!

Dealing with your feelings

The first emotion most people feel (once they've managed to accept that the test result is genuine) is a sense of absolute euphoria. Finally, after all this time, you've done it. The veil of gloom that has soured everything in your life will slowly rise, at last you will be able to move on, and the family experiences that you have dreamt of for so long can now be part of your world too. It's a moment of sheer elation, but it is often followed very swiftly by a host of other emotions, as the joy is eroded by anxieties about the future.

A positive pregnancy test is usually the start of a journey, but when you've already had a long trek to get to this point, it feels as if you ought to have arrived. Finding yourself beset with a plethora of new worries that almost inevitably accompany pregnancy can be a surprise – you may wonder whether your body is really capable of carrying a baby after such a long wait, whether you will miscarry, or whether there is something wrong with the baby or the pregnancy. You are so used to having your hopes shattered, and so used to dealing with disappointment, that you may find yourself focusing on the things that could go wrong and mentally preparing yourself for the worst. The best piece of advice I was given about this came from one of the midwives who looked after me throughout my pregnancy, who explained that just because I'd had problems getting pregnant, it didn't mean that I had to have problems *being* pregnant. It's absolutely true, so try to keep this in your mind.

One worry that can become overwhelming for women who've had difficulty conceiving is the fear of miscarriage. You have probably heard that miscarriage is more common after fertility treatment, but it is important to keep this in perspective, as it doesn't mean that fertility treatment itself makes you somehow more likely to miscarry. Instead, this is linked to the fact that women who have treatment tend to be older, which increases the risk, that they often know they are pregnant much earlier than women who conceive naturally so will be aware if they have a very early miscarriage, and that they may have gynaecological conditions that can make them more likely to miscarry. There is no reason to assume that you are more at risk of losing a baby just because you've had fertility treatment, and although it is probably inevitable to worry about this to some degree, try not to let it dominate your pregnancy.

People can react in very different ways to the news that they are finally expecting, and some women feel a sense of ambivalence, or even negativity, despite the fact that they have been trying for a long time. You may have got to a point where you stopped believing that it could ever happen for you, and finding yourself faced with the reality of pregnancy you may start to panic, wondering quite what you have let yourself in for and whether you truly wanted this to happen. This may just be part of a protection mechanism if you are finding it difficult to believe that your luck has finally changed, or it may be an indication that there are underlying issues that have not been addressed. If you are feeling panicky, or unsure that this is what you wanted, it may be a good idea to make an appointment to talk to a counsellor, as it can help prevent fears from building up.

If you've had treatment to get pregnant, you are likely to have been making frequent visits to your clinic during the weeks leading up to your pregnancy, and you will have been very closely monitored. Once you've had a positive pregnancy test, it will be a couple of weeks before you have your first scan. This can seem a long gap when you are used to such regular appointments, and people do sometimes wonder why they can't have a scan right away, but at the time of the positive test, the embryo is still too tiny and doctors would not be able to get much useful information about the pregnancy from scanning at that stage. By six or seven weeks, there is a visible embryonic presence in the womb, and the clinic will be looking for a heartbeat.

The expert view
Mollie Graneek, specialist fertility counsellor

'I think people get to the stage where they are almost expecting their treatment not to work – and then when it does, it is quite a shock to them. It's a very perplexing dynamic as there aren't just two people making this baby, there's a whole clinic of specialists, and so in some ways they feel quite exposed. It's almost like a sense of abandonment when it works, because there is somebody holding their hand at every stage of the way in that earlier phase and all of a sudden there's nothing.'

The signs of early pregnancy

The first and most important thing to say about the signs of early pregnancy is that you are unlikely to have any if you find out that you are pregnant very early on. When you've tried to have a baby for a long time, and especially if you have been through fertility treatment, you will be testing long before most women would if they had got pregnant naturally, and the signs of early pregnancy won't usually appear until a little later.

There will probably have been many months in the past when you have wondered whether you could possibly be pregnant, and have perhaps felt a little nauseous or tired. Women who've spent some time trying to get pregnant tend to be experts on the early signs of pregnancy. When we first started trying to have a baby, every time my period was due I would start to question whether I was feeling a bit sick, or whether my tummy looked very slightly rounder than usual. Even as I became less and less optimistic about ever getting pregnant, I still spent the last few days before every period imagining symptoms. In reality, it would be most unusual to start experiencing dreadful morning sickness or peculiar food cravings when you were just four weeks pregnant, so you shouldn't worry if you don't have any of the symptoms you have spent so long imagining.

Some signs of very early pregnancy are similar to those you may feel when you are pre-menstrual and they may include:

- Needing to urinate more frequently
- Tiredness
- Nausea and sickness
- Sore or swollen breasts
- Tender or sensitive nipples
- Heightened sense of smell
- Odd tastes or cravings

When I was pregnant for the first time, I didn't have any signs at all for the first few weeks and was desperate to start feeling sick or craving pickles with jam just to confirm that I was really pregnant, and so I was absolutely delighted when I first started to feel slightly nauseous.

Do remember, it's the positive test that tells you that you are pregnant, not any other signs.

The first scan

If you've got pregnant after treatment at a fertility clinic, you will usually be asked to go back to the clinic for a first scan when you are around six or seven weeks pregnant. The pregnancy dates from the end of your last period rather than from the moment of embryo transfer, so this first scan will be two or three weeks after the positive test. It is a big moment, as this will be the first time that you get to see your baby, and the weeks between the positive result and the first scan can seem interminable. I was sure I would feel a lot more confident about the pregnancy after the first scan, and every day in the time leading up to it seemed to last for about a week. I was terribly nervous by the time we went in for the scan, and desperately worried that something might have gone wrong in the interim and that it would reveal an empty womb.

The scan is carried out by vaginal ultrasound, just like the other scans during your fertility treatment. My husband and I were both on tenterhooks as we waited to see the scan picture emerge, and then completely stunned when the doctor pointed out a little pulsating bean-shaped dot on the screen and explained that the pulse was our baby's heartbeat. It is amazing to get to see your baby at such a very early stage of development, and I think we need to see this as one of the odd pluses of having a fertility problem. You may even be given a printout of the ultrasound scan to keep – your first baby picture!

The second scan

There is usually a second scan which is carried out at around eight or nine weeks. By this time, your bean should have grown to look slightly more like a prawn and may be developing bud-like fledgling limbs, although you are unlikely to see much more than a slightly larger pulsating blob on the screen. It may still feel like very early days, but if all is well at this scan, you have already jumped lots of the hurdles along the way towards a healthy ongoing pregnancy.

Once you reach this point, you are ready to be discharged by the fertility clinic and move into the care of maternity services. Although I'd spent years dreaming about leaving the fertility clinic behind for good, I suddenly felt quite anxious about losing the safe reassurance of the regular appointments and checks, and I wasn't sure I felt ready to deal with the world of antenatal care outside. When I mentioned this to the doctor at my last appointment at the clinic she cheerfully told me, 'You're not special any more, you're just like everyone else now.' It was meant to be positive and reassuring, but actually I didn't feel remotely like 'everyone else'. I knew I was still an anxious fertility patient on the inside, and worlds away from other pregnant women who hadn't had any trouble conceiving.

The expert view

Tarek El-Toukhy, consultant in reproductive medicine, Guy's and St Thomas' Hospital

'All clinics will usually do a first scan between six and seven weeks. There is not much point in doing a scan

continued

---

before that, as you wouldn't be able to see the three things that we are looking for – a healthy gestational sac, a yolk sac and a heartbeat. We also carry out a second scan two weeks later. If everything is normal at that second scan, the patient can be further reassured because at each step the miscarriage risk declines. At the first scan, the miscarriage risk is about, say 15 per cent, but by the next one it has gone down to between 7 per cent and 10 per cent, and by the next scan it will be just 2 per cent to 3 per cent. Sadly, sometimes between the first and second scan the pregnancy development can stop, so it is hugely reassuring to see that the pregnancy is growing normally. Depending on the skill of the sonographer, it is also sometimes possible to tell a bit about the probable progression of the pregnancy, even at this early stage. They may be able to measure the heart rate, and by this stage we could see if a baby was small for age and not developing well.

'We normally discharge people to maternity services after the second scan at eight or nine weeks, but we are very aware that the first antenatal scan is not until 12 weeks, so that does leave about a month between the two. Some patients do feel anxious, and if they do, they can contact the clinic and see if they will do another scan. We would stress that this is not at all necessary, it is a luxury, but if a patient is really anxious, if they have any bleeding or any odd symptoms, or if the symptoms they'd been having suddenly disappear, they can contact the clinic. We don't want to leave our patients in limbo.'

What can I do to try to ensure I have a healthy pregnancy?

When it has taken time to get pregnant, you will want to do all you can to try to make sure that your pregnancy goes well. Many women feel that they should wrap themselves up in cotton wool during early pregnancy, and they worry endlessly about what they should and shouldn't do. I think most of us would probably like a long and very prescriptive list of exactly what we ought to do or should avoid, but really most of it is common sense. There is absolutely no need to retire to bed at this stage unless your doctor has specifically told you to do this for some reason. Generally, it is far better to be up and about and doing things. If something makes you feel anxious, uncomfortable or concerned, don't do it – not because it will make a difference to the outcome, but because it may leave you fearful and worried.

Smoking

Most smokers give up if they are having problems getting pregnant, as smoking is linked to infertility. You really shouldn't smoke when you are pregnant, and if you have given up, this is definitely not the time to consider starting again. Smoking during pregnancy can restrict your baby's oxygen supply, there is a greater risk of miscarriage and stillbirth and your baby is more likely to be born prematurely and to have a low birth weight.

If you are a smoker and you are finding it really hard to give up, you should cut down as much as you possibly can right away. Your doctor will be able to offer help with giving up smoking, and you should take advantage of this.

Alcohol

Current medical advice is that you shouldn't drink alcohol at all during pregnancy and that if you do continue to drink, you should limit yourself to one or two units of alcohol once or twice a week. This advice has been questioned by some academics who claim that there is simply not the medical evidence to back up suggestions that a moderate intake of alcohol during pregnancy could cause problems. Obviously, you don't want to do anything that would put your baby at any kind of risk, but there really is no need to worry or to feel guilty if you enjoy an occasional glass of wine during your pregnancy.

Drinking excessively during pregnancy has been linked to low birth weight, heart defects and learning and behavioural disorders. In severe cases, babies can suffer from fetal alcohol syndrome, which leads to facial deformities, poor growth and all kinds of mental and physical development problems, but this only occurs when women are drinking quite considerable quantities of alcohol while they are pregnant.

Folic acid

You should have been taking folic acid during the time that you have been trying to get pregnant. Some women who have been trying to conceive for many years stop taking folic acid because it can start to feel like a daily reminder of what they are unable to achieve. Don't worry if you haven't taken folic acid in the run up to pregnancy, but do start again right away. Folic acid can help prevent neural tube defects such as spina bifida, which usually occur during the first 12 weeks of pregnancy.

Pregnancy multivitamin

Taking a daily pregnancy multivitamin pill is not going to do any harm, and may fill in any gaps you aren't covering in your diet. There is a wide range of multivitamin pills specially designed for pregnant women on the market, and they will also contain your daily dose of folic acid.

Healthy eating

There's no need to become manic about what you eat, but it is important to follow the basic rules on healthy eating at this time. You may find that you don't like certain foods that you usually enjoy and that you develop some food obsessions or cravings. People sometimes report all kinds of strange food fads during pregnancy. There are some foods that you should avoid, such as soft unpasteurised cheese and raw meat (details on page 46), and your doctor or midwife will give you a list of foods you shouldn't eat during pregnancy.

Exercise

Women often worry about over-exerting themselves in early pregnancy, and feel that perhaps they should be resting all the time, but in fact there is no need not to take normal exercise when you are pregnant. Of course, it is sensible to avoid anything excessively strenuous, but there is no advantage to taking to your bed. See Chapter 2, page 48 for more about exercise during pregnancy.

Relaxation and stress relief

Most women feel anxious during early pregnancy, and if you can do anything to help yourself feel more relaxed this will help. Often women are keen to continue with any complementary therapies they've had while they were trying to get pregnant, but you should talk to your practitioner about what might be suitable for you in early pregnancy before going ahead with any of these. Whether you've tried them before or not, meditation and visualisation are techniques that you may want to consider, as they can be very calming. It's important to find something that suits you, and it may be as simple as some early nights with a good book, but do try to ensure you think about your emotional well-being as well as your physical health, and don't feel guilty about devoting time to looking after yourself.

The expert view

Tarek El-Toukhy, consultant in reproductive medicine, Guy's and St Thomas' Hospital

'The reason most clinics don't give women advice on what they can and cannot do in early pregnancy is because, to be honest, we don't know. Anything that is sensible is going to be all right, so it is fine to do gentle exercise – to do the shopping, to go walking or swimming; however we don't advocate doing anything

continued

excessive or any kind of strenuous exercise – do you really need to do an hour-long exercise class? It's better to wait until we know what is going on and how the pregnancy is progressing. If you develop any spotting, any bleeding, any unexpected pain or unusual discomfort, then contact the clinic or doctor, and slow down and rest. It's common sense rather than science. I know people worry about what they can and can't do at this time, but it's an area where science can be a bit inadequate and you should follow your common sense.'

When should you tell people you are expecting a baby?

Some people are so excited when they finally get a positive pregnancy test after years of trying that they can't resist telling everyone right away. Others would rather take some time to let the news sink in and to share the excitement with their partner and close family before starting to tell other people. If your friends and family were aware that you were going through a treatment cycle, they will be longing to know the outcome and you may have to share your news much earlier than you would have chosen. This can feel slightly uncomfortable if you've told a wider circle of friends and acquaintances about your treatment, since in normal circumstances you might not have chosen to tell so many people about the pregnancy at just four or five weeks. It can feel as if even

the decision about when to tell others has been taken
away from you because of your fertility problems, and
that it is another way in which infertility can continue
to make you different. If you've told a small group of
people about the treatment, you can share the news with
them, but explain that you'd rather they didn't tell
everyone else right away.

We only told the close circle who had known the details
of our treatment cycle that we had finally been successful.
I didn't want to start telling everyone because it felt too
early and too uncertain, but as it was the only thing I
could think about all day, every day, it was sometimes
hard to be with people I knew well but not quite well
enough to want to share the news with them so soon. I
ended up avoiding some social events for a while because
I felt that it must be obvious from my face alone that I
was so much happier after years of going around under
a cloud of gloom; however, I was also still worried about
letting myself really start to believe I was properly pregnant and might be having a baby in eight months.

At the time of my first pregnancy, I was working as a
producer at Channel 4 News. I had to tell my boss that
I was pregnant, as she'd agreed to me taking some time
off for the IVF treatment cycle, but I'd said I didn't want
anyone else to find out until I felt more confident about
the pregnancy. I had my 12-week scan at a leading fetal
medicine unit, and I knew that the main consultant there
had been in the news that day, commenting on a story
about early pregnancy. We were sitting waiting in a long
queue for our scan when I spotted ITN's health reporter
and her camera crew arriving at the other end of the

corridor, ready for an interview with the consultant. I sank into my seat, wondering whether there was any way they might not spot me, when I heard one of the crew say, 'Oh look, Channel 4 News are here already!' They came bouncing up and I had to explain that actually I was pregnant and was waiting for a scan, not to do an interview. I felt extremely anxious about having to tell them before I went in for the scan, as if it might somehow affect the outcome, but it was clear that I wasn't going to be able to keep my pregnancy under wraps any longer. In fact, once I'd been for the scan and had seen my baby moving about, it felt quite liberating to be able to tell people and to end the secrecy which had enveloped our lives during the years of trying to conceive.

If you've built up a network of friends who were also experiencing fertility problems and going through treat-ment, it can be very difficult to know how to deal with telling them when you discover you are pregnant. You have probably been in the position yourself in the past where one of your group has announced a pregnancy, and you recognise that the happiness you feel for a friend is overshadowed by a degree of jealousy, and by a sense of fear that you are a step closer to being left as the only childless member of your circle. You know how it feels, so try to be as sensitive as you can in the way that you tell other people. If you've been attending a support group, it may not be appropriate for you to go back to announce the news and it would probably be better to call or email. If you've been using an online support network you should make sure you use the right part of the forum to tell others, as some people find pregnancy announcements very painful. You may still feel that you need support at this time, but it is important to appreciate that although you are feeling anxious and tentative about your pregnancy, to those who haven't yet managed to conceive you have already achieved what they most want.

There are separate areas on many of the fertility websites for women who are pregnant after fertility problems, and it can help to be in touch with others who are in the same position. Although there are countless sources of support, information and advice for pregnant women, you may not feel that they meet all your needs, and it is often useful to talk to other people who are pregnant or have children after fertility problems, as they will understand your perspective. There is also a charity, ACeBabes, just for those who are in this position, which offers support and advice.

'ACeBabes was set up in 1998 after I had my son, Adam. When I went back to the fertility clinic where I had my treatment to show him to them, I felt out of place, as if I didn't deserve to be there because of all the people in the waiting room who were still trying. It was difficult to let go of a place that had been my life for the last year or so, where all my hopes and dreams had risen and fallen. I felt I needed to share how I felt and so ACeBabes was conceived. A group where the issues of becoming pregnant after years of being infertile could be aired, where the prospect of further treatment could be discussed and where you could be honest and make friends who knew exactly what you had been through. Now the group is a national charity with a growing membership both in the UK and overseas.'   *Helene Torr, Founder, ACeBabes*

The booking appointment

Once you are in the normal maternity care system, the first stage will be a booking appointment, which is carried out by a midwife or a doctor. This is a fairly detailed meeting, which usually takes at least an hour, and the midwife will run through the details of your medical background and your general health. You will be given advice and information about nutrition and exercise during pregnancy, and about the antenatal care and tests that you will have further down the line.

There may also be some advice about breastfeeding and maternity benefits, and the midwife may want to discuss your options for planning your labour and where to give birth. I was surprised to be asked questions about my birth plan at this first booking meeting; I was still trying to believe that I was really pregnant, and hadn't ever dared to venture as far in my thoughts as considering actually giving birth to the baby. What's more, I had resolutely avoided other women's conversations about midwives, epidurals, Caesarean sections and all related topics for so long that I hadn't the least idea about what sort of birth I was anticipating, and it felt far too early to be even thinking about such things, let alone making any kind of plans.

It's a good idea to take a pen and paper to this appointment so that you can jot down anything you might forget, and making a list of questions you want to ask in advance can be helpful. Don't ever worry about asking too many questions, as this is what the booking appointment is for. The midwife or doctor may be aware of your fertility history, but if they don't know about the treatment you've had, you should be honest at this stage. Sometimes people feel that they don't want the stigma of being a former fertility patient, but in fact it can mean that you will be treated with a little extra care and attention, which certainly won't be a bad thing – another of those unexpected bonuses from having had fertility problems!

It can be hard to relax at this time and you may feel you'd like a scan every day to reassure you that everything is all right. Try to remember how you dreamt about being pregnant and how you would have felt if you'd known you would eventually get to this stage – this is the culmination of all that you have been through and now is the time to try to relax and enjoy it.

Lisa's story

Lisa and Adam had been trying to have a baby for six and a half years. They'd tried IUI and Lisa had suffered an ectopic pregnancy and lost one of her Fallopian tubes before she conceived her daughter.

'I'd given up doing pregnancy tests because it was just so upsetting, but my period was late and I still had a few tests left, so I thought I'd do one. My husband was working away and it just came up really faint. I get asthma and I was so shocked that I had an asthma attack, almost a panic attack, because I just couldn't believe it. This was at about 11 at night, and I had a couple more tests in the cupboard so I did another two and they both came up positive as well. I thought they must be from a dodgy batch of testing kits because they were old. I was awake all night till the supermarket opened at six in the morning, and then I went to get another one. That was positive as well – and then I had to wait all day for my husband to get home from work. I wasn't going to tell him right away, but he could see it on my face.

'Luckily the hospital booked me in for an early scan because I'd had an ectopic pregnancy before, so it was confirmed then that the pregnancy was where it should be. I was just stunned really – I couldn't believe it. I was excited, but also really anxious, and every day I was expecting that my period would start. I wanted to have a scan every day, but once you're in the system you are just normal. It was really difficult – there are massive gaps between appointments even though I did have a few more scans because of my previous ectopic. I didn't feel at all the same as other people who were pregnant. I did NCT [National Childbirth Trust] antenatal classes and everyone there had just conceived really quickly. Although we got on fine, I did feel a bit removed from the situation. On the antenatal form where it asked for any other information I said 'Yes, IUI' – I wanted everyone to know what I had been through.

'I just kept expecting things to go wrong. I think I was in shock for the whole nine months. For me, I felt it would be a miracle if I did have a baby at the end but I wasn't expecting it, definitely not, not after so long. For the first five months I was just expecting to have a miscarriage. It was only in the last two or three months that I started to think it was possibly going to happen.'

CHAPTER 2

Pregnancy

It will take time, but your pregnancy should gradually start to feel more real as each week passes and your bump begins to grow and to show. You may still feel in limbo, however; as if you are no longer infertile but not entirely 'normally pregnant' either. It can be difficult to deal with this, or to know how to explain it. When you tell people that you are pregnant, their joyful reactions can seem at odds with your own natural sense of caution. Of course, there are some people who are able to put the past behind them as soon as they discover they are pregnant and to move on, but for most of us, the long journey leading up to that positive test does leave an imprint.

I read a suggestion that it might help if you did something to celebrate, to mark the end of your fertility problems and the move on to the start of a new phase of your life. This is a lovely idea as you have waited so long to be pregnant and achieving your goal seems to deserve some joyful recognition. Having said that, I appreciate that for some couples, celebrating at such an early stage might not feel right. No matter how much reassurance you receive, it can seem as if the long-awaited finishing line you've always imagined you'd reach once you got pregnant has suddenly jumped nine months further ahead.

It may help in early pregnancy if you can try to remember how happy you imagined you would be if you ever managed to get pregnant. You may not have a baby yet, but you are on your way towards your goal and for most of us this is further than we have been before. You may feel uncomfortable dancing for joy, but try to relish your growing bump and enjoy the feelings you have yearned for. When you are pregnant, every day can seem to go so slowly as you wait tentatively for each stage of pregnancy to pass, setting your sights on the moment at which you will finally have to believe that you are going to have a baby. For some people, this comes fairly early on in the pregnancy, but for others it isn't until the birth itself that they can allow themselves to accept that they are about to become parents. When you look back on your pregnancy, it will seem to have whizzed by and you will strive to remember what it was like to first feel your baby move, to see your body changing and to walk around with an ever-larger bump. It is a shame to let anxiety dominate every moment of your pregnancy, so do try to allow yourself to take pleasure in the pregnancy you have waited so long to experience.

Care during pregnancy

For most women, your main point of contact during pregnancy will be your midwife. There will be a series of appointments, which may take place at home, at an antenatal clinic, at a doctor's surgery or at the hospital. Apparently – and possibly rather alarmingly for former fertility patients – most women have up to ten antenatal appointments during pregnancy, which works out at just over one a month. I know I would probably have been reassured by weekly appointments throughout my pregnancy, and I did worry during the long waits between my visits to the midwife, fearing that I had every pregnancy complication imaginable. If there were any signs that you were at risk, or had a more complex pregnancy, you would be seen more often, and anyone who is expecting more than one baby will have more regular checks. Having normal, albeit alarmingly long, gaps between appointments is a sign that everything is going well, so try to keep that in mind.

Although you want to stop feeling different now that you are finally pregnant, there is sometimes an underlying sense of panic: a feeling that your luck at finally getting a positive test result can't possibly continue, that you don't really deserve to be pregnant, or have any confidence in your body's ability to carry a baby. I had got used to being a fertility patient, and to all the special care that came with it. I was almost cocooned in a life that was focused on trips to the fertility clinic. I knew the staff, and they knew every detail of our long journey to pregnancy. Now, suddenly, I was expected to be just another expectant mother when I felt like a fraud and was still consumed with anxiety.

If you are feeling worried, don't be afraid to say something to your doctor or midwife. Although some may be more understanding about what you have been through than others, there is a general recognition that you are likely to need more reassurance if it has taken you some time to get pregnant. If you know it would help you to be seen more frequently, do ask about this, as it is often possible.

The expert view
Professor James Walker, Royal College of Obstetricians and Gynaecologists

'Obviously, people who have an IVF pregnancy have probably been trying for a number of years to become pregnant, and this pregnancy is very precious to them. Their anxiety levels about what is going to happen to them and what is going to happen during their pregnancy are different from that of an 18-year-old who comes along with a first pregnancy. There is a lot of psychological reassurance required because they will be more anxious if the baby is not moving properly or if there are slight concerns about a rise of blood pressure. For any problem in pregnancy, they will have heightened anxiety because it is so precious to them, and any worry will be more worrying. A lot of it is just tender loving care – they're probably going to be seen more often, just to make sure everything is going OK. These things are not really required medically but are there to be reassuring and to make sure all is well.'

Pregnancy checks

....

As we have seen, you will have regular checks throughout your pregnancy to ensure that everything is going as it should. Most of these will be with a midwife unless your pregnancy is deemed to be high risk, and remember that having had fertility problems or treatment doesn't automatically make your pregnancy high risk. When you've been through a lot of treatment to get pregnant, you may feel that you want to see a consultant every time you have a check, but this really isn't necessary and a midwife is often better equipped to look after you during your pregnancy.

The midwife will check the baby, feeling your bump and listening to the heartbeat, and will also make sure that you are OK. You will usually have a blood pressure and urine test to make sure that there are no signs of raised blood pressure, infection or pre-eclampsia. Sometimes women who are very anxious can feel that their midwife or doctor brushes over their concerns, not really appreciating how much a small rise in blood pressure or a throwaway comment about your bump being a bit small or large for dates can send you into a panic. For the professional, your pregnancy may seem completely ordinary while for you every moment of it is infused with significance. Don't let this prevent you from mentioning any worries or concerns, or any symptoms that you aren't sure about, as it is important to get reassurance; however, try to remember that there is no reason for fertility problems to lead to pregnancy problems.

The expert view

Manjit Randhawa, matron, high-risk midwifery team, St Thomas' Hospital

'Sometimes a woman is labelled as a complex, high-risk pregnancy as soon as she is pregnant after fertility treatment. Straightaway, either the health-care professional or the couple themselves see it as high-risk pregnancy. We find that frustrating because we do feel women will miss out, especially on things like antenatal classes. If you try to normalise your pregnancy, you have a positive experience in your pregnancy and a positive outcome.

'The role of the midwife is to be the woman's advocate and do her antenatal checks. Anything outside what is perceived as normal is handed over to the obstetrician. If fertility treatment leads to a single pregnancy and the pregnancy is absolutely normal then in that case it is midwifery-led care – they would see a consultant obstetrician maybe once, and then that's it. If it is straightforward and normal she does not need to be referred to an obstetrician for her antenatal checks, antenatal classes and the management of her pregnancy right up to labour.'

Not feeling 'properly' pregnant

You may have all the signs of pregnancy, you may have had a scan and seen the baby, your bump may be starting to show, and yet you somehow don't feel 'properly' pregnant. If you're still struggling to believe that you are pregnant, the idea that you will have a child in less than a year may be completely unfathomable. I'm sure pregnancy feels incredible to any expectant mother, but when you have waited a long time the whole thing can seem quite surreal.

I used to turn up at antenatal classes feeling as if I wasn't quite meant to be there, as if I had somehow managed to sneak my way into a private club I didn't have the right qualifications to join. I often used to sit next to a woman who was expecting a baby a week before mine was due and would look at her bump thinking that it looked more 'real' than mine. It wasn't until we'd both had our babies that I discovered that she'd had fertility problems too, and her son was an IVF baby. Not everyone wants to talk about their past problems once they are pregnant, and it may well be that some of the other women you are assuming have achieved their pregnancies naturally and easily have gone through just as much as you to get to this point.

Pregnancy isn't always easy

When you've spent years dreaming about being pregnant, you've probably managed to whitewash over most of the less pleasant aspects in your head. I know I had visions of myself wafting about with a neatly rounded bump, blooming rosy cheeks and a permanent smile. The reality was somehow far less wholesome. My pregnancy began with a rash of spots and I spent most of it looking lumpily overweight rather than glowingly pregnant.

Many women really suffer during pregnancy. You may experience nausea and sickness, tiredness and exhaustion, backache, leg cramps, indigestion, heartburn, flatulence, bloating, constipation, headaches, varicose veins, swelling of the ankles, faintness, breathlessness, forgetfulness, nasal congestion, bleeding gums and haemorrhoids. When you list the possible symptoms, it's hardly surprising that it isn't always the blissful experience you may have imagined.

The expert view
Mollie Graneek, specialist fertility counsellor

'Sometimes once people achieve the so-wanted pregnancy, it is wretched. They are sick and tired but feel they can't moan because people are going to be unsympathetic. They can feel a bit lost and isolated in that wretchedness that sometimes accompanies pregnancy – but they don't dare complain for fear that something awful is going to happen because they've been miserable.'

You are also likely to feel some emotional changes during your pregnancy, and many women find that they feel vulnerable or tearful at times. In early pregnancy, women often experience mood swings and you may get irritable or panicky. When you combine the hormone-induced mood changes with the huge rush of emotions that engulf you on discovering you are finally pregnant after trying for some time, it is hardly surprising that it can be more difficult than you had anticipated.

What makes all this particularly challenging for anyone who has been trying to get pregnant for a while is the feeling that you can't possibly complain about any of it, no matter how tired or sick or uncomfortable you may be. Most pregnant women don't have any qualms about expressing some ambiguity about their situation now and again, but you are only too aware of how desperately you wanted this, of how fortunate you have been to get pregnant. You may feel you have no right to express any kind of doubt, uncertainty or discontent about your pregnancy, no matter how rough you feel, because you have always imagined that you would relish every moment if you ever got lucky. All of these things make your pregnancy very different from those of most women who have conceived naturally without any trouble.

'I had a terrible pregnancy. I was sick all the time and I felt so bad. You hear about people having morning sickness and you think it's just when they wake up, but I felt sick all day. I was so tired and then my feet swelled up and my blood pressure kept going all over the place. It wasn't at all like I'd expected, but you can't ever say you feel bad because you know how much you wanted to fall pregnant. I just kept thinking it was because my body wasn't meant to have a baby and it couldn't cope.'   *Hayley*

Dealing with your anxieties

One of the reasons for offering more monitoring during pregnancy to women who have had previous fertility problems is the recognition that they may feel anxious about the pregnancy. Most pregnant women worry about their babies to some degree, but fears and concerns are often heightened by the knowledge that you might not be able to conceive again. In retrospect, I'm surprised that my son doesn't suffer from some kind of sleep disorder as I used to start to worry whenever he was still for too long and would prod my stomach until I felt him moving. The poor child was probably desperate for a proper sleep by the time he was born.

Don't worry about expressing your concerns to your midwife or doctor. It is better to be reassured than to get yourself into a panic, and they are used to dealing with problems in pregnancy.

'Looking back on my pregnancy, the IVF overshadowed the whole experience. I was just so anxious throughout it all, so worried about everything and it wasn't helped by the long gaps between appointments. During the treatment, I'd been so used to being seen all the time and having that constant reassurance. It destroyed the pleasure of finally being pregnant, because although I did try, I couldn't just relax and enjoy it. One of the reasons I really want another baby is because I'd make the best of it if I ever get pregnant again.'   Jess

Is it my baby?

One fear that certainly is unique to people who've had assisted conception is an underlying concern about the possibility of the baby they are carrying not being theirs. Not everyone thinks about it, but I know at the back of my mind, there was an unspoken sense of unease about the fact that my eggs and my husband's sperm had been in a laboratory for days where anything could have happened to them. There have been occasional shocking news stories about mix-ups in laboratories: the black twins born to a white couple, the couple whose last remaining embryo was transferred to the wrong woman, the eggs fertilised with the wrong man's sperm. When these awful mistakes occur, they have such a huge impact that many fertility patients are left with a nagging sense of disquiet about the possibility of human error in the laboratory.

I think I was more concerned about the possibility of some kind of mix-up when I was pregnant with my second IVF baby, perhaps because we'd had a frozen embryo transfer which meant that the embryo had been in the care of the clinic for months rather than days. I hadn't been aware of feeling unduly worried about it until my sister came to visit just hours after my daughter had been born. She burst out laughing as she walked into the room, and said she couldn't believe how much her new niece looked like me. I was surprised to feel a sudden rush of relief at the recognition that this obviously was our baby, that there hadn't been a mistake – she was my daughter.

I spent time in fertility clinic laboratories watching embryologists at work when I was researching *The Complete Guide to IVF*, and I was struck at the time by how rigorous they were about double-checking the labels on every petri dish before moving anything from one place to another. Some clinics now have elaborate electronic or bar-coding systems in place to prevent any mix-ups, while others employ double-witnessing procedures where two embryologists check the details before sperm, eggs or embryos are moved in the laboratory. There are such good systems in place that it is highly unlikely that errors will occur, and on the rare occasions that mistakes do happen, they are usually discovered immediately, which makes it even less likely that you could possibly be pregnant with the wrong embryos.

For couples who have used donor eggs or sperm, there is often an underlying unease about what the baby will be like when it is born. People don't always admit to this because they find it hard to talk about, and they may feel it is something they ought to have come to terms with before they went through treatment rather than during pregnancy. Once people have had their child, they don't always want to say that they were worried that the baby might be somehow freakish or abnormal. It's not a shallow or silly worry. It is only natural to feel some anxiety and uncertainty about this, and knowing that it is a common worry may help. You can find more about this in Chapter 11 on donor families.

Fertility treatments and your baby's health

There have been some studies in recent years linking IVF and/or ICSI to genetic abnormalities or birth defects in babies, and these have greatly worried some prospective parents. It is important to keep this in perspective. While it is true that there have been studies suggesting an increased risk after fertility treatment, this is a small increase in a tiny risk and in real terms the chances of your baby being affected are extremely low. The vast majority of babies born after fertility treatment are absolutely fine, and multiple birth is more of a risk after IVF than this.

The cause of this slight increase in risk is not clear, but researchers aren't assuming that it is necessarily anything to do with the treatment itself, as parents who've had fertility treatment are often older, are more likely to have multiple pregnancies and may have fertility problems which affect their sperm and egg quality.

Saying goodbye to your fertility network

Pregnancy can be quite a lonely time for women who've experienced fertility problems. Many of us build up networks of friends who are going through the same thing when we are trying to conceive unsuccessfully. When your existing friends all seem to be getting pregnant and having babies, their lives change and it can feel as if they are leaving you behind as they move on to a new stage of life. In the circumstances, your new-found fertility friends can become very important to you in a relatively short space of time, and yet it is often hard for these sometimes extremely close friendships to endure once one of you is pregnant. You know how it feels when one of your network of fertility friends announces a pregnancy, and how the happiness you feel for them is tempered by a sense of panic that yet another person has moved on, and by the fear that you may never get to that stage yourself. You know only too well that the last thing they need is to be faced with your growing bump and your insecurities about pregnancy, but having to leave those good friends behind can be a real wrench, especially as you probably feel a need for all the support you can get in early pregnancy.

Sometimes these friendships will survive one of you getting pregnant, particularly if a friend has a positive test not long afterwards, but this isn't always the case. It is important to recognise that sometimes particular relationships fit at a particular stage in your life, and that a very close friendship which occurs when you are thrown together by a set of circumstances won't always last when circumstances change.

Changing relationships with friends

Until I got pregnant, I'd never really understood the phrase 'being in the club', which is sometimes used to describe pregnancy. It was only when I suddenly acquired a whole new group of friends who had young babies within weeks of announcing my pregnancy that I realised it really did feel as if I had joined some kind of club. It was most noticeable at work, where there seemed to be an unspoken bond between the mothers in the office. Colleagues I'd only had a passing relationship with would stop and chat at my desk, telling stories about their own pregnancies and babies. Women I'd barely known before lent me books about pregnancy and birth, and even maternity clothes. I was really touched by the kindness people were showing, but at the same time it seemed ironic that there was a sudden swell of support once you finally got pregnant, and yet there had been so little during the years of trying unsuccessfully to conceive.

The male perspective

In theory, pregnancy should bring the two of you together as you anticipate the birth of your longed-for child, but during pregnancy the attention is focused on the female who is carrying the baby and it can seem to be a rather one-sided experience. When a woman is pregnant, she is very conscious of all the physical changes that are going on in her body and she gradually begins to build up a bond with her unborn baby. Sometimes, men can become slightly detached from what is happening and may even harbour a sense of resentment that they are being left out of things. At the same time, women sometimes resent the fact that their male partners don't appear to be taking the pregnancy sufficiently seriously.

Once you've reached the point of a successful ongoing pregnancy, the male perspective is often that you both ought to be able to relax a little and enjoy things. Remember that it may be far easier to take this attitude when you are watching the pregnancy progress from the outside. Women can feel a huge weight of responsibility as their bodies are charged with the physical care and welfare of the child during pregnancy. Women who've had fertility problems often have very little faith in their own bodies, and may worry that they won't be up to the task of nurturing the growing baby. It can be really helpful to have a calm and collected partner if you are permanently anxious, but that has to be accompanied by a sense of understanding. It is important to try to adopt a sympathetic attitude, no matter how irrational your female partner's fears may seem, as women are awash with hormones during pregnancy and being tearful and worried now and then is par for the course.

The absolute key to ensuring relationship problems don't arise during pregnancy is to make sure you communicate with one another properly. Talk about any concerns and anxieties and listen to your partner's point of view. At this time, you will both be very focused on the pregnancy but it is a good idea to make some time for things that you enjoy that aren't baby-related, whether that might be going out for a meal, to the cinema or the theatre or for a walk or day trip somewhere. Once your baby comes along, you won't have much time to do things alone together and although you may feel now that you are looking forward to that, it's a good idea to ensure you do all you can to shore up the foundations of your relationship, as life with a new baby can be testing, no matter how much you wanted a family or how well you think you get on.

Having a healthy pregnancy

You will be bombarded with advice about what you should and shouldn't be doing when you are pregnant, and there's no shortage of advice about how to keep healthy. On the whole, it's a matter of common sense. There's no need to mollycoddle yourself for nine months, however tempting that may be, but equally it isn't worth risking doing anything that is going to worry you.

Official advice plays it safe and it can feel as if you have a long list of rules, relating to diet in particular, that are never to be broken. Your midwife or doctor will give you full details of everything you shouldn't eat, but the basic forbidden foods are:

- Soft cheeses, such as Camembert or Brie (cottage cheese is fine)
- Blue-veined cheeses, such as Stilton or Roquefort
- Any kind of pâté
- Raw meat or poultry – when cooking poultry or meat make sure that it is properly cooked all the way through
- Unpasteurised dairy products
- Raw eggs or products made with raw or partially cooked eggs, such as homemade mayonnaise
- Pre-prepared salads
- Ready meals or reheated food unless they have been thoroughly cooked and heated right through
- Unwashed fruit or vegetables
- Raw shellfish

These rules about what not to eat are mainly to help avoid any risk of food poisoning, of listeriosis (a type of infection caused by bacteria in certain foods), or of toxo-plasmosis (an infection caused by a parasite that is most often transmitted by contact with cat faeces or raw or uncooked meat). You should also remember to always wear gloves when you are gardening, and if you have a cat, try to get someone else to change the litter tray or ensure you wear gloves to do this.

We had been invited to supper by some neighbours during the early weeks of my first pregnancy, before we had told anyone that we were expecting a baby. I was horrified to discover that the salad we'd been served contained tiny lumps of blue cheese, which I didn't notice until I'd eaten one. I spent the rest of the evening inwardly fretting that I was going to lose my baby thanks to one minute piece of blue cheese. In fact I was fine, and it is important to remember that while it is generally good advice to avoid certain foods when you are pregnant, both listeriosis and toxoplasmosis are really quite rare and the guidelines are cautionary, so if you happen to eat some forbidden food, you don't need to panic.

It goes without saying that you should avoid any kind of recreational drug during pregnancy, but you should also be careful with some common prescription and non-prescription drugs. Check with your midwife before taking any kind of drug, and always remind the doctor that you are pregnant if you are prescribed anything.

It is impossible to avoid all environmental pollutants entirely for nine months, unless perhaps you go and live in isolation on an island in the middle of nowhere, but it does make sense to try to limit your exposure to toxic substances wherever you can. Things such as garden pesticides or powerful domestic cleaning fluids often carry warnings about their potentially harmful contents, and you should avoid these wherever possible.

A fit pregnancy

During pregnancy, you should try to keep active, as it is good for you and your baby, and apart from anything else, it will help during labour if you are fit. Women who've taken time to get pregnant are sometimes more cautious about exercise in pregnancy, fearing that they might do something to put the pregnancy at risk. I was so anxious in my first pregnancy that I became obsessed with the idea that I shouldn't go swimming in case another swimmer accidentally kicked me in the stomach and hurt the baby! The fact that this had never happened during all the years that I'd been swimming didn't stop me seeking advice about it from my doctor, who reassured me that she had never ever come across a case of anyone having pregnancy problems due to swimming. Please don't let my neurotic worries put you off swimming, as in fact it is an ideal form of exercise during pregnancy, along with any other gentle activity. You may find special antenatal exercise classes at your local leisure centre – yoga and aqua aerobics are often particularly popular. These can be very helpful as they also offer the opportunity to meet other pregnant women and exchange tips and advice.

Complementary therapies

If you used any complementary therapies regularly when you were trying to get pregnant, you may want to continue with them during pregnancy. They may help reduce stress and keep you calmer and more relaxed, while also allowing an opportunity to indulge yourself a little. Do tell your therapist that you are pregnant, and they can tailor your treatment to make sure it is appropriate. Of course, not everyone likes complementary therapies and they can be costly, too. If you want to get some of the benefits without the cost, you can always give yourself a spa session at home and do your nails, put on a face mask and sit in a warm bubbly bath!

Antenatal screening

You will be offered routine screening tests during your pregnancy on top of the normal blood and urine tests. These screening tests are to check that your baby doesn't have chromosomal issues such as Down's syndrome. The tests may include a blood test or a scan or both. It is important to be aware that they don't give definite answers as to whether your baby has a problem, but merely offer an assessment of risk, and you don't have to have the screening tests if you'd prefer not to. If the risk looks high, if you are older or have a family history of genetic conditions, you may be offered chorionic villus sampling or an amniocentesis. These are more invasive tests that give a definite picture.

Chorionic villus sampling (CVS) is usually done between 10 and 13 weeks, and tests for genetic or chromosomal disorders. It involves taking a small sample of the cells from the placenta which can either be done by inserting a needle through the abdomen wall or by putting a thin tube through the cervix. Amniocentesis is carried out after 15 weeks of pregnancy and a needle is used to pass through the abdomen and take a sample of the amniotic fluid. These tests are carried out only when there are reasons to think that there may be a higher than average risk of chromosomal abnormalities, and both carry a small risk of miscarriage.

When we went for our 12-week scan, I was hoping to leave feeling reassured that everything was OK. Although I was nervous, I was looking forward to finally being able to tell people other than our close friends and family that we were expecting a baby and anticipating that we would be able to allow ourselves to really enjoy the pregnancy for the first time. Our delight at seeing our little baby looking like a real person for the first time, waving his arms and appearing to clap his hands, was soon dissipated by the radiographer who told us that the scan showed a higher-than-average amount of fluid behind the neck. Our risk of having a Down's syndrome baby was instantly recalculated from low to high for my age, and I was advised to go for a further scan at a specialist centre where they would also be able to carry out CVS.

It felt once again as if our chances of being happy and relaxed about the pregnancy had been snatched away, as suddenly there was a whole new set of things to worry about. I started frantically reading up about Down's syndrome and CVS, and realised that given our level of risk, the chances of losing a possibly healthy baby after CVS were greater than the chances of having a baby with Down's syndrome. We had already decided that we wanted our baby regardless of whether he had Down's, so there seemed to be little point in going ahead with an invasive test just to be sure one way or the other. Although the likelihood of having a Down's baby diminished as the pregnancy went on, the risk still lurked in the back of my head throughout the pregnancy. I know that for many women, getting a certain diagnosis would have outweighed any potential risks, but the perspective is sometimes different when you don't know whether you would ever be able to conceive again.

The fear of pregnancy loss

Concerns about the possibility of having a miscarriage dominate many pregnancies conceived after fertility treatment. It is a shame that so much time is spent worrying about this, but it is perhaps inevitable that the fear of losing a baby is particularly acute when you don't know if you will be able to get pregnant again. It is true that there is an increased risk for some people who are pregnant after fertility treatment but that is related to the fact that they tend to be older, that there is a higher chance of a multiple pregnancy, and a higher risk for those with some of the conditions that cause fertility problems, such as polycystic ovary syndrome.

It can be particularly difficult to be calm about the risks if you've already had a miscarriage or ectopic pregnancy in the past, and there is more detailed advice on this in Chapter 3 on miscarriage. In general terms, although it is important to be sensible during pregnancy, most women who've had trouble getting pregnant are likely to be doing everything they can to ensure that they don't encounter any problems. Try to remember that if a miscarriage is going to happen, there is really nothing you can do to stop it occurring, but equally you are extremely unlikely to do anything during pregnancy that could cause a miscarriage.

The expert view
Ruth Bender-Atik, The Miscarriage Association

'The bottom line is that a lot of miscarriages are caused by things that are beyond our control, so although there may be things that one can do to increase the chances of a healthy pregnancy and minimise the risk of miscarriage, people generally know what they are. It's all about cutting out cigarettes and alcohol, avoiding blue cheese and unpasteurised dairy products, avoiding toxoplasmosis and trying to be calm and relaxed. Even if you do all of those things by the book, you can still miscarry. There may be things that you can do to reduce your risk but even if you do them that's not a guarantee.'

A high-risk pregnancy

Some pregnancies after fertility treatment will be deemed as high-risk, perhaps because there is more than one baby or because of a medical or physical condition that could cause complications. Some conditions that can develop during pregnancy, such as pre-eclampsia which is associated with high blood pressure and protein in the urine, can lead a pregnancy to be reassessed as high risk. If your pregnancy is deemed to be high risk, you will be seen more frequently, but it doesn't necessarily follow that there will be problems with your pregnancy or the birth.

You may feel as if your fertility problems are still haunting you if you have a high-risk pregnancy after finding it hard to conceive. It is incredibly stressful to be constantly worried about whether things are going to be all right, and you may not feel you can enjoy pregnancy or feel confident that you will actually become a parent. It can put a great strain on your relationship too, which will have already been tested by fertility problems.

High-risk pregnancies are closely monitored, and you will have more appointments with more senior medical staff and more scans. Of course, it is worrying to know that your pregnancy is considered to be risky, but you can be reassured that any potential issues should be swiftly picked up as you will receive more tailored care.

Antenatal classes

I was desperate to go to antenatal classes, as all of my friends who'd had babies used to talk about their NCT classes, which came to epitomise the other world I couldn't enter when I was trying unsuccessfully to get pregnant. I registered for classes as soon as I'd had my 12-week scan and was terribly disappointed to discover that they didn't begin until you were about 30 weeks pregnant. It is worth going to any kind of antenatal class you are offered during pregnancy, as it is really helpful to meet other pregnant women and to share experiences. I did feel slightly awkward at first in antenatal classes, as if I didn't have the same right to be there as everyone else. Not everyone feels this way, but if you do, don't let it stop you going to classes or joining in with things once you are there, as they can be really helpful.

I also did a pregnancy yoga class when I was pregnant for the second time, and I found that really worthwhile. We focused a lot on keeping calm and breathing, and I do think it helped me to be more relaxed when I went into labour. There are all kinds of different pregnancy groups you could consider, from hypnobirthing or active birth classes to aqua-natal (that's exercises in water) and parentcraft. Go along to any kind of class that appeals to you, as it will not only help you prepare for birth and becoming a parent but it will also be a good opportunity to meet other pregnant women and will help to normalise your pregnancy.

Getting ready for your baby

If you've worried about tempting fate throughout your pregnancy, you may not have wanted to start buying things for your baby. While other mothers-to-be are decorating nurseries and bulk-buying nappies when they are just a few months pregnant, you may have felt uneasy about getting confident too early on. Parents who have waited for pregnancy don't always entirely manage to believe that they are ever going to have a baby, even when faced with a huge bump, and you may feel you want to wait until you are sure everything is going to be all right before you start shopping.

Of course, you should be guided by your own feelings and do what suits you, but at the same time, for most prospective parents, getting ready for their baby is something that is fun and enjoyable. Finally, it is your turn to go into the baby shops you have spent the last few years taking long detours to avoid, you can pick the tiny outfits you like and contemplate the merits of different types of cots, buggies and car seats. You don't have to do things too early, but at the same time, you don't want to leave it so late that you are rushing around in a mad panic at the last minute, which can make the whole thing become a desperate chore rather than a pleasure.

Louise's story

Louise and her partner, Joseph, had four cycles of ICSI before they finally discovered she was pregnant. Louise was 16 weeks pregnant when we spoke.

'I think it is different being pregnant after IVF than when it is a natural pregnancy. With IVF, as each cycle fails it gets tougher, and having a family seems further and further out of your grasp. You start wondering whether it is ever going to happen for you, it seems to elude you more and more with each disappointment.

'You have this fantasy idea about how excited you will be if you ever get pregnant, and how you will run and tell everybody, but we were just really scared. I kept thinking that someone was going to take it away from us, and I still feel that at 16 weeks. I still feel that somebody is going to snatch it away, because it has been so wanted. I know it's not rational, but when it actually does work, you are even more worried that you might be tempting fate by getting too confident somehow. You feel so damaged by the whole thing and so frightened.

'Obviously, parents, close friends and colleagues knew what we were going through. It's really hard because they know you are going to be testing. When people have been so supportive throughout, to shut them out and not tell them when you get the result feels wrong. We were trying to keep it quiet and were avoiding other people because they were going to ask when we were next going to do IVF and then of course we couldn't make things up, you have to tell them straight then. We avoided them because I couldn't think of anything else to say apart from that I was finally pregnant but that we didn't want to tell them that because we weren't over that first 13 weeks. There was just that whole business of feeling that it could go wrong and you might never get pregnant again. There are still friends of mine who are quite good friends but who don't know — either because it hasn't been the right time to tell them or because I want to tell them face to face.

'We are expecting twins and I felt a bit robbed because I had it in my head that once we'd got to 13 weeks we'd be in with a good chance. But then we were told that there were all these other risks for us from 16 weeks onwards because they are identical twins sharing a placenta — it was a whole different ball game. We had just been starting to feel a bit more confident and then it all got crushed again.

'There is this risk of twin-to-twin transfusion syndrome, where one twin gets all the blood. It can be very dangerous so they are checking me for that. I have two-weekly scans, but they are saying that it is looking good because of the way that the babies are lying and the way they're growing. It makes me feel a bit confident — but every time I feel more confident it's as if something comes along to take it away again so you are very fearful of feeling confident.

'I'm delighted and very excited about having twins, but I do sometimes wonder why it always has to be complicated — why I can't just be like a normal mum and put all that IVF stuff behind us. The identical twin thing happens more frequently because of IVF, and probably wouldn't have happened if we had got pregnant naturally, because it doesn't happen so much then. Everything seems to keep going back to the IVF.

'I know everybody who is pregnant has anxieties, and you don't want to constantly make out that you and your pregnancy are more special than the next person's, but I do feel a bit like that. In my close family, there is that acknowledgement that you've got to be extra careful because if anything happened it would be so difficult to start again, it's an almost unspoken acknowledgement.

'I manage a team, and before I told them I said to my manager that I would have to say it was all very touch and go, but he said, "No, you don't have to say that at all, just tell them you are pregnant with twins." They were all so excited and it made me think that was how it should be – I shouldn't have to tell people my news with a proviso that it might all go wrong. It was nice to just go with the moment. Other people have a spontaneity about it which I don't feel I can have. Part of me is holding back, and I think, *When can I relax? When can I enjoy this?*

'You begin to believe that you are like the kid with your nose against the glass of the sweet shop. You feel that only other people can have these things, that somehow you are excluded from them, that you don't deserve it, that you are not part of that society that is going to be a mum or have a family. It's very hard to see that you've crossed that line and that you are actually in the sweet shop now. Even buying maternity clothes took me a while to get my head around because I felt I wasn't entitled to do that.

'I know I need to try not to be so anxious and worried. I said to my husband that there does have to come a time when we accept that these babies are going to arrive and start making arrangements for them. We will have to set a date in the diary where we will mentally make a decision that they are actually coming and that we are not going to be holding back on this level.'

CHAPTER 3

Miscarriage

For women who are expecting a baby after experiencing fertility problems, the fear of miscarriage can sometimes overshadow the entire pregnancy. It's probably only natural to worry when you have waited so long to get pregnant, but it is a shame to let that fear taint what ought to be a time of joy and happiness.

Try to remember that having had fertility treatment in order to conceive doesn't increase your chances of losing your baby, and that if you are following the sort of sensible advice for anyone in early pregnancy, you are unlikely to be doing anything that is going to cause a miscarriage.

Pregnancy loss is far more common than most of us realise, and about one in four pregnancies will end in miscarriage. It's not an easy statistic for anyone who has had fertility treatment, and the risk is greater as you get older, but remember that the majority of women who've had a miscarriage do go on to have a successful pregnancy. I know it can be difficult and most of us are anxious and concerned, but spending the early days of your pregnancy worrying is not going to reduce your chances of having a miscarriage.

What can I do to prevent a miscarriage?

Women often assume that there are things that they can do in early pregnancy that can either cause a miscarriage or prevent one. In reality, there is little that you can do that will make a difference, and you can't really prevent a miscarriage if it is going to happen. Of course you should follow sensible advice about eating healthily, exercise and lifestyle, and you should steer clear of the food you are told not to eat during pregnancy, make sure you keep fit without doing anything too excessively strenuous and avoid cigarettes and alcohol. If you've been trying to get pregnant for a while, it is likely that you will be sticking to these guidelines anyway.

Sometimes women feel that they should do as little as possible during the first few months, because they are constantly worried that everything might be putting their baby at risk. You really don't need to take to your bed or to stop leading a normal lifestyle just because you are pregnant. There is no evidence that this will reduce your risk of miscarriage, and emotionally it may make things worse, as you will be constantly focused on the possibility of a negative outcome.

The expert view

Mollie Graneek, specialist fertility counsellor

'I think there is a myth with IVF that you will in some way induce a miscarriage if you don't rest up once you've had the embryo transfer, which is nonsense. Trying to tell people to carry on as they normally would falls on deaf ears because they feel that they need to wrap themselves up in cotton wool. They fear something happening and then if something does happen, they blame themselves. They tend to reproach themselves for something that they have done. It has been proven that there is nothing that people can do that will make a difference.'

What are the signs of miscarriage?

When it has taken you a while to get pregnant, you may be hypersensitive to any twinge or ache during early pregnancy. There are sometimes cramps and mild pain in pregnancy, and it is easy to assume that these must be a sign that something is going wrong. Of course, if you have severe cramping pain you should seek medical advice right away, but more gentle aches and pains are often just part of pregnancy as the ligaments that hold the womb stretch to accommodate a growing baby.

There can also be spotting or light bleeding, and again it is important to try to keep in mind that this doesn't necessarily mean that anything is wrong. Some women have what is known as 'implantation bleeding', which occurs when the embryo implants into the wall of the womb, or they may have some bleeding at around the time that a period would have occurred. If there is any bleeding, especially if it is accompanied by pain, you should take this seriously and seek medical advice, but don't immediately assume that you are losing the baby. Your doctor would normally offer an ultrasound scan and may also do another pregnancy test to check what is happening.

'A few weeks into the pregnancy, we were due to go away and I started bleeding one night. I bled quite a lot and at that point we thought that was it. We phoned the hospital helpline and they said it could be implantation bleeding, that we shouldn't panic and to go to the unit in the morning. So we drove in the next morning and they did an emergency scan. It was the first scan that we had and we saw a heartbeat, but I still didn't believe we would see it all the way through.'

Diana – who had a successful pregnancy after this early scare

What happens during a miscarriage?

Bleeding and cramping are the most common signs of miscarriage, and it is important to seek medical advice if you experience any kind of bleeding or severe stomach cramps. Most miscarriages occur during the first trimester, or the first 12 weeks of pregnancy. Sometimes there is severe bleeding and all the tissue from the womb is discharged. This is known as a complete miscarriage and if this happens you will not need any further treatment.

Sometimes when a woman has a miscarriage, not all of the placenta, sac or embryo is discharged and there may be continued bleeding or pain. This is known as an incomplete miscarriage, and it may be necessary to clear the womb to ensure there is no risk of infection. Doctors may allow you to wait for this to happen naturally, or you may have medical treatment or a minor operation to ensure that all the tissue has gone from the womb.

Occasionally, a woman is unaware that the pregnancy has been lost as there have been no outward signs that the fetus has died or stopped developing. This is known as a missed miscarriage, and is sometimes only discovered during a routine check up. If this happens, you may miscarry naturally shortly afterwards or you may need a minor operation to clear the womb. Missed miscarriages usually occur in the early stages of pregnancy, but can be extremely distressing. It generally only happens because there is something wrong with the baby which would have prevented normal development.

What causes miscarriage?

For anyone who has lost a baby, the first thing you want to know is why it happened and how you can stop it ever happening again. It is often hard to pinpoint the exact cause of an individual miscarriage, and most women who lose a baby will never know why it happened. Pregnancy loss is not usually investigated after a first miscarriage, which can be very hard to bear if you are desperate to find out what went wrong. The reasons for not investigating are based on the fact that miscarriage is so common that often no reason can be found, and that most women who've had a miscarriage will go on to have a successful pregnancy.

It is important to stress again here that it really is most unlikely to be anything that you have done that has made a difference. Women often go back over everything they've done during their pregnancy and become convinced that it is their fault because they drank a glass of wine, lifted some shopping, didn't get enough rest or got stressed at work. None of these things will make you miscarry. Generally, when a pregnancy is lost it is because there is something wrong with the fetus, and it is not your fault.

Although it can be hard to work out why an individual miscarriage might have occurred, there are some common causes:

- In as many as half of all early miscarriages, the embryo can't develop properly because there is some kind of abnormality in the chromosomes. These chromosomal problems are more common in older women, but there's no reason to assume that this will happen again in a future pregnancy if it happens once.
- Women who have certain hormonal problems, such as polycystic ovary syndrome, are more likely to miscarry. If you have irregular periods caused by hormonal imbalances, this increases your risk of miscarriage.
- Another common cause of miscarriage is anti-

phospholipid syndrome. Women who have this have antibodies in their blood that can cause blood clots. It is thought this may stop the placenta forming properly or prevent an embryo implanting, and it can lead to recurrent miscarriage.

- Some infections can increase the risk of miscarriage, such as listeria, chlamydia and uterine or vaginal infections. Although most normal infections would not have an effect, if you have a very high temperature this can lead to problems.
- Large fibroids, which can cause infertility, may also increase the risk of miscarriage in some cases.
- Problems with the cervix can be a cause of later miscarriage, as a weak cervix may start to open when the baby gets heavier.
- Smoking increases the risk of miscarriage, as does heavy drinking (see also page 20).

Age and the risk of miscarriage

Women are not always aware of how age impacts on the risk of miscarriage. We are born with a finite supply of eggs, and as we get older our eggs get older too. No matter how young we look or feel, or how fit we keep ourselves, there's nothing we can do to prevent our eggs from ageing. As our fertility declines more sharply from the age of 35, so our risk of miscarriage rises. For women between the ages of 40 and 44, there is a 51 per cent chance of losing a baby, and the risk continues to rise rapidly for women over this age. Doctors sometimes find it hard to tell women that their age is the most likely reason for losing a baby, as they know there is nothing anyone can do about age-related pregnancy loss. Of course, it is upsetting to think that your age gives you a higher miscarriage risk, but it is probably better than worrying that you must have done something wrong.

Investigation after miscarriage

It is only when women have been through the trauma of recurrent miscarriages, which generally means three or more, that they will be referred for investigations into why they have lost their pregnancies. This can seem incredibly tough for women who don't get pregnant easily in the first place, and sometimes there is some flexibility if you've had fertility treatment and have miscarried for a second time. Even for women who do manage to get some specialist help, there is often no cause found for the miscarriage, but research has shown that just being reassured that you are being cared for more closely during the pregnancy can improve outcomes.

The expert view
Ruth Bender-Atik, The Miscarriage Association

'It would be extremely rare to have an investigation after a first miscarriage. Even if you wanted to pay somebody privately, they would probably try to persuade you to

continued

try again, because the overall risk of having a second miscarriage is really no different from the risk of having a first.

'Although the general rule of thumb tends to be that investigations will be offered after three consecutive miscarriages, there are places where you will get them after two, and if there have been later losses and women who have age and fertility problems, that might swing it. It is absolutely understandable why you would want to know why you have miscarried, but you need to understand that at least half of the couples who have the investigations won't come out with an answer.'

Ectopic pregnancy

An ectopic pregnancy occurs when the embryo implants itself outside the womb, usually in the Fallopian tube. People sometimes assume that this can't happen after IVF or ICSI, as the embryo has been transferred back into the womb. In fact, although it is quite rare, the embryo can sometimes move from the womb into the tube. It happens most often in women who have had an ectopic pregnancy in the past, those who have blocked or damaged Fallopian tubes and those who have a history of pelvic inflammatory disease.

If you have an ectopic pregnancy, you will have a positive pregnancy test. The embryo may not survive for long, but if it continues to grow in the tube it will soon become painful as it stretches the tube walls. There may also be bleeding or spotting, but this is not usually like a normal period, as the blood is often dark and watery. An undiagnosed ectopic pregnancy can be very dangerous, as the embryo may cause the tube to rupture, causing severe pain and bleeding.

Women who've had fertility treatment usually have early scans and sometimes blood tests to confirm the pregnancy, and this can help diagnose an ectopic pregnancy. If a pregnancy test is positive, but there is no sign of an embryo in the womb, this can be an indication of an ectopic. An ectopic pregnancy is never going to be viable, but early diagnosis and treatment is essential to ensure that there is no danger of the Fallopian tube rupturing. Sometimes it is possible to treat an ectopic pregnancy without taking out the tube, if it is discovered early on, but it is often necessary to remove it entirely.

Having an ectopic pregnancy can be a traumatic experience, particularly for women who have taken some time to get pregnant in the first place. You may feel you aren't sure you want to go through treatment again, and it often takes a while to recuperate both physically and emotionally. Allow yourself time to recover. Having had an ectopic pregnancy in the past does put you at greater risk of having another, but you can be reassured by the fact that you will be monitored closely after future successful fertility treatment to check that there is no danger of this.

The expert view

Tarek El-Toukhy, consultant in reproductive medicine, Guy's and St Thomas' Hospital

'A blood test can raise suspicions of an ectopic pregnancy, but you would need to do serial tests in order to be sure about this. If the HCG level doesn't rise as expected, then the pregnancy probably isn't viable. It may be non-viable but in the right place, or it can be non-viable and growing in the tube as an ectopic pregnancy. We carry out serial blood tests routinely for patients who've had a previous ectopic to both confirm the pregnancy and exclude the risk of an ectopic.'

Stillbirth

If you lose a baby after 20 weeks, this is classified as a stillbirth. As with any pregnancy loss, it is not always clear why this has happened. It is more likely to occur in a multiple pregnancy, and most often happens when the mother is apparently healthy and the pregnancy is close to term. It is important to keep the risk of stillbirth in perspective, as it is a rare occurrence.

Vicky's story

Vicky had an early miscarriage after her first IVF cycle, so she and her partner, Alex, were overjoyed to discover she was pregnant with twins after her second attempt.

'When I got to week 20 and had my scan and everything seemed OK, I decided to start getting organised. I knew that the twins were boys. Twin two would constantly kick me all the time and move about, so he became known as Cheeky Charlie, twin one was James. We took all the classes that the hospital offered including a very good multiple-birth class, which was great to meet other women who were having twins.

'I had no immune system while pregnant. At around 20 weeks I had the flu, and I had to have antibiotics to get rid of it. Once I got over that bug, I got a chest infection and then I got flu again. The bugs were endless. I had no energy and could not get about much because I was huge.

'When I was 35 weeks, I vomited all night and into the next day. I have never been so ill. I got the doctor out to see me. He was so concerned he admitted me to hospital to get rehydrated. I was put on the maternity ward and I was placed on a drip. They checked the boys, and at this stage they could only find one heartbeat on the listening machine. They weren't concerned, as they thought that one twin was hiding behind the other. I was in hospital overnight. In the morning they again struggled to get the machines to pick up both heartbeats. I was not overly concerned as I could still feel movement, or what I thought was movement.

'They wanted to check by scanning me, so I went to the scan department and I wandered in relaxed. Once the scan started, I could see the midwife going through all the points with James, then she moved on to check Charlie. I remember her turning to me and saying she couldn't find twin two's heartbeat. I could not believe what she was saying. Another one of the nurses came in and she confirmed her findings.

'We were moved into another room and we both just cuddled each other and cried our eyes out. We were totally shocked. We could not believe what we were being told. I had considered all the problems with pregnancy and childbirth; however, I never really thought about stillbirth.

'I remember our doctor coming in to speak with us and she was going through all the options with us. She organised for me to go in two days later for a section when she would be at work. I remember sitting in the chair crying for two days, I kept blaming myself for the loss. My mind went all over the place at that time.

'I was taken in to get the drugs administered in my back, which did not work, and eight attempts later I said 'just knock me out'. Once I was brought around, I saw James and he was a wonderful little boy. I could not believe I had done it; we had a lovely little boy – he was mine. I was then asked if I wanted Charlie bringing in. I could not do it.

'I spent five days in hospital. It was Christmas and we were having the worst weather for years. On Christmas Day, I met Charlie. We had him blessed. It was awful looking at him lying so still on the bed and I had James in his cot just next to the bed sleeping soundly. It was a very sad strange day, not a normal merry Christmas. I never imagined I would suffer the loss of one of my children in my lifetime.

'When I got home I think in the early days the nights

were the worst, when I was up alone, trying to feed James I would think about Charlie and how it would be if he was there. We had Charlie tested to see if there was a reason for what happened but we had no answers. As time went on I didn't need answers as much, I just accepted that you can't change it and there's no reason to dwell on it.'

The emotional impact of miscarriage

Losing a baby when you've already experienced fertility problems can be totally devastating. Miscarriage is difficult for anyone, but it feels like a double blow when you don't know whether you will be able to get pregnant again. Women in this situation often feel very isolated and lonely. Although other people may tell you that they have miscarried in the past and want to reassure you that you will go on to have a successful pregnancy, they don't appreciate how it feels when you can't just go off and get pregnant as soon as you want to. Friends who are still going through fertility problems and treatment may feel that you are somehow better off than they are because you have at least managed to get pregnant, which is one step further down the fertility road. This is not always helpful, and you need to allow yourself time to go through the grieving process.

The expert view
Ruth Bender-Atik, The Miscarriage Association

'People are hugely distressed. If you finally get pregnant and then have a miscarriage it can be devastating – it is a double blow. Dealing with all of this at once makes it very hard to bear. A lot of miscarriages are caused by things that are beyond our control and generally speaking if you are going to miscarry, you will miscarry. The risk is complex because it depends on factors including age and the number of previous miscarriages, and also fertility history as well as some medical history. The rate of miscarriage after treatment is not associated with the fertility treatment, but obviously if you've got a multiple pregnancy then you automatically have a higher risk of miscarriage whether you've had IVF or not. There does seem to be a link between time taken to conceive and miscarriage, in other words if it took you longer to get pregnant and there is possibly an underlying sub-fertility then that is linked with a higher rate of miscarriage. That's true whether this was an IVF pregnancy or a natural pregnancy.

'There is some evidence that men's age makes a difference independent of the age of the mother, but for the most part we tend to be looking at women because we are born with all the egg cells we are ever going to have. The older we get, the older they get and some of them will be less than perfect, which can mean it takes longer to conceive or that there is a higher risk of a baby with chromosome abnormality, and some of those will miscarry.'

Counselling

Whether you've opted to have counselling for your fertility problems or not, it may really help to see a counsellor after a miscarriage. Sometimes there is a temptation to jump into more treatment as soon as possible and to try not to think about what has happened, but it can help if you acknowledge and accept your feelings of grief, as this will help you to move on. If you can see an accredited fertility counsellor, they will be an expert in this area and able to understand all the complex emotions involved.

Complementary approaches

As I explained in Chapter 2, people often think of complementary therapies when they are trying to find help to get pregnant, but they may not think to turn to them after a miscarriage or unsuccessful fertility treatment. In fact, complementary therapies can be particularly helpful at crisis points as it's not just the treatment itself that can help, but also the counselling element. A complementary therapist will be able to devote some time to listening to you, to talking to you about how you feel and to helping you prepare yourself for whatever you decide you want to do next, whether that is more treatment, some time off to think or moving on to a new path.

The expert view

Gerad Kite, acupuncturist

'Miscarriage is probably one of the most distressing things because in the existing medical system people are not even looked at until they've had three miscarriages. Doctors may be naturally empathetic or have natural skills with people, but they are not really trained how to be useful in a very proactive way to people who are simply distressed about something. If you give a patient comfort and confidence that they can achieve what we are trying to achieve, that in itself can make a dramatic difference to them. Hopefully, we actually strengthen the system if it is to do with a weakness so that they don't miscarry but it is also about how to cope on an emotional level. So acupuncture is not just about sticking needles into people, it is a about a relationship with the practitioner and feeling really listened to and looked after, and that's a very important part of the care.'

Recovery

You will need time and space to recover after a miscarriage, and you should not expect yourself to be able to get on with life as normal right away. If you appreciate this and allow yourself time to grieve for your loss, things will get better, although of course this will take time.

Everyone reacts differently and people's feelings about their loss and how they deal with it will not be the same.

Some people can take enormous solace from the fact that they did manage to get pregnant, and are able to see this as something positive – a step further down the line, and one that not everyone who has fertility problems will ever reach. This may be true, but for many other women suggesting that they might draw some comfort from the fact that they got pregnant is absolutely the worst thing that anyone can say and this is an equally valid and understandable reaction.

Talking about what has happened is often good therapy, and the fertility and miscarriage support organisations listed at the back of the book will be able to help with this if you don't feel comfortable talking to friends or family. It can be incredibly helpful to talk to someone else who has been through a similar experience; however, some people really don't want to talk to anyone about what has happened, and it is absolutely fine if you feel that way. You have to do what feels right for you.

It is important to do all you can to look after yourself at this time. Take some time off work, maybe go away for a few days. Spoil yourself and do some nice things that you enjoy if you feel able to. Go to see your complementary therapist, or to a spa or beauty salon if that's your thing. It may help if you try to focus on getting fit and well, and having some kind of action plan for the future can be beneficial to some women. Above all, be kind to yourself and understand that it is going to take a while for you to feel in control again.

You may find that holding some kind of ceremony to acknowledge your loss is helpful, perhaps planting a tree or plant in your garden, or in a forest or wood.

The grief you will be feeling can be totally over-whelming, and it is easy to get submerged by it. These small steps to helping yourself may be enough to ensure that you keep your head above the water until the raw emotions gradually begin to subside.

Fertility treatment after a miscarriage

Your consultant will let you know how long you need to leave before trying fertility treatment again after a miscar-riage, but do ensure you allow yourself some time to recuperate mentally as well as physically. Sometimes people want to start again as soon as they can, but you will need space to grieve for what has happened, and it may help if you have built up your mental strength in order to feel prepared for more treatment.

The treatment process itself can feel more fraught after losing a pregnancy because each step is just another along a path you've already travelled. Having a good crop of follicles, a successful egg collection, fertilised eggs and healthy embryos may not make you feel as positive as you would have done before your miscarriage. You are more likely to have successful treatment if you've been pregnant in the past, but if it doesn't work, you may begin to wonder how much more you can put yourself through and to feel that you will never have a family. It can be particularly difficult to deal with an unsuccessful cycle if your finances are tight and if you aren't sure when, or even whether, you will be able to pay for more treatment.

Even when fertility treatment is successful, you may not feel that you can celebrate after your previous experience. People often find it hard to enjoy any pregnancy after fertility treatment, but this will be exacerbated if you have lost a baby in the past. You may feel particularly anxious until you are past the stage of your previous miscarriage. Try to remember that having one miscarriage doesn't make you more likely to have another, and that most people do go on to have a successful pregnancy after miscarriage.

Sophie's story

Sophie and her partner, Nick, had already suffered three miscarriages before beginning IVF. After an unsuccessful first IVF cycle, their joy when Sophie finally became pregnant was short-lived, as antenatal testing at three months showed that the baby had a very serious genetic disorder. Sophie and Nick were told that they would have to terminate the pregnancy. A year later, Sophie had a third IVF cycle, and discovered she was pregnant again.

'When we got pregnant, I didn't even allow myself to believe it was positive. For me, it was hard to get over that sense of gloom. I do look back on it as a very lovely time – but in the back of our minds there was always the idea that it might go wrong and we mustn't tempt fate. We kept setting milestones – that we'd be happy when we got through the 12-week scan, and then we would be happy when the baby was viable, and happy when we got through the next scan. We did it in chunks in the way that we'd done the IVF.

'I have memories of it being a beautiful time because he was healthy and I was healthy, but I didn't have a baby shower, I didn't go out shopping with my friends, I didn't test drive a push chair. I didn't buy anything – I couldn't face it because I thought, *If he dies, I'll have to take all this stuff back to the shops and say that my baby has died and you'll have to take it all back.* I remember going to my first pregnancy yoga class, and most of the others were second-time mums, or a lot more pregnant than me, and I felt like a complete fraud. You could barely see my bump. They were bulk-buying cheap nappies, and I was thinking, *But you've got five months of pregnancy left, what if your baby dies?* I didn't buy anything, not a thing until the last week. I only did it when I had to, because my mum made me.

'So many times I'd had midwives' appointments and then had to cancel them because I'd miscarried, so I told my doctor I'd arrange a midwife's appointment myself after the 12-week scan. I couldn't bear to have to send back another pack of NHS maternity forms.

'I didn't believe that we would come home with a live baby when I went into hospital to give birth. I was so used to babies dying. The birth was horrible. It all went horribly wrong. My waters broke about six days before he was due and I went into hospital and was induced. He was back to back [in a posterior position, where the baby is facing outwards with his head pressing against the pelvis] and stayed that way, and I had forceps and a Caesarean. It wasn't exactly the roses around the door, but Nick held him for the first 40 minutes and they have a wonderful relationship. I don't think I had postnatal depression and I don't think I had a problem bonding, although it took me a long time to believe that he was here for good. I was slightly detached.

'I realised that I never held any babies other than my own, because for ten years I had avoided other children. I cut myself off from babies and pregnant women, and I carried on doing that. I could hold my own son and look at him, but I didn't dare hold anybody else's because I was still in that mindset that I was an infertile woman.

'I wasn't able to feel positive until our son was about nine months old. I don't know what made things change but I remember when he was nine months I woke up one morning and I thought, *I really love you*, and it was the first time I'd really, really felt it – maybe the first time I'd allowed myself to feel it. He feels like my son now, and I don't feel as if he's not going to be around any more.'

CHAPTER 4
Birth

Pregnancy can seem a very long and drawn-out business, but in the last few weeks you should start to feel more relaxed as you are finally heading for the home straight. It may only be now that you can really start to believe that you are going to be giving birth and will soon have a baby of your own.

By this stage, you will have decided where you want to have your baby and you will have discussed the sort of birth you would ideally like. Although there is no reason for the way in which a baby was conceived, or the length of time it has taken you to get pregnant, to influence your plans for the birth, you may find that this does shape your views. Be guided by your own instinctive feelings about this, don't feel pressured into plans that don't feel right for you and remember that there are no right or wrong ways to give birth.

Birth plans

You will be asked for your thoughts about the sort of birth you'd like fairly early on in your pregnancy, and will usually draw up a birth plan with your midwife or doctor in the last trimester. This will include details of the sort of birth you would like and the pain relief you want to be offered, if any. You can even include details of which position you'd like to be in when you give birth and who you'd like to be with you.

Don't worry too much about your birth plan, as it is only a plan, and labour is never predictable. First babies often take longer to be born, and you may find that you change your mind about the sort of pain relief you'd like during labour itself, or that circumstances dictate that you have a different type of delivery. I found the idea of birth planning quite hard to get to grips with as it seemed to start at such an early stage that I wasn't entirely confident about being pregnant, let alone thinking as far ahead as giving birth to a baby. I had spent so long avoiding people's birth stories that I had no idea what sort of pain relief I wanted or whether I wanted fetal monitoring, and it was quite hard to think about these issues in any kind of logical way because it didn't come naturally to assume that I was going to get as far as labour. Even if you feel this way, it's important to devote some time to your birth plan because it is your chance to express your thoughts about this, which you may not be able to do when you are in the middle of labour.

Don't feel you haven't done things properly if you don't end up following your birth plan, as it's really not the most important thing at this stage, and it's very common for people to have a completely different birth from the one they've described in their birth plan. I said I wanted to try to have a drug-free natural delivery if possible for my first baby, but I ended up having my waters broken by a consultant and an oxytocin drip and epidural, which certainly hadn't featured in my birth plan. Sometimes people who have taken time to conceive are worried that they will have particular problems giving birth too, but there is absolutely no reason for this. It's true that there are more Caesarean sections for IVF babies than for naturally conceived babies, but this isn't due to the IVF itself but has more to do with the age of the mother and related medical conditions.

Preparing for the birth

As you approach the last few weeks, you should be able to relax and start to get ready for your baby. If you have felt wary about buying clothes or nappies, now is the time to enjoy getting everything ready. You may seem to need a bewildering array of stuff, and you could spend a small fortune on equipment, so do talk to other people who have children about what was useful and what wasn't. If your friends all have older children, they may have baby things that they can lend you, too. It can feel very strange to find yourself purchasing all these unfamiliar items and spending time in shops you've conspicuously avoided for so long, but try not to let your past experiences overshadow what ought to be a time of eager anticipation.

As you approach the last few weeks, make sure you have the basics that you will need for yourself as well as your baby. It's often the practical but dull things that get overlooked, like stocking up your kitchen cupboards and freezer. If you have the energy, cooking some meals and freezing them will be an absolute godsend once the baby comes along, as you are unlikely to find much time for cooking.

You will also need to prepare yourself for labour, getting together a hospital bag with everything you might need. Your midwife will be able to help with what you should take, and you will get advice on this in antenatal classes too.

These last few weeks of pregnancy often feel rather strange and drawn-out, but it can be a lovely, peaceful time if you have stopped working. Try to relax, get as much rest and sleep as you can and don't feel you have to dash around doing things. You will be large and you will be tired, and it's a good time to enjoy indulging yourself a little as there will be little time for this in the months ahead.

Aiming for the perfect birth

There can be a lot of pressure on women about the type of birth they have. We are often told about the negative effects of certain types of pain relief, or of certain types of delivery. Many women, not just those who have had problems getting pregnant, end up feeling that there is some kind of ideal birth that they should be aiming for, and then feel that they have failed if they don't achieve it. This can be particularly acute when you have already experienced the distress of feeling that your body is letting you down by having problems getting pregnant. Don't forget, the definition of an 'ideal' birth can be very different from one woman to the next; while one person might actively seek an elective Caesarean feeling that this would be safer, another might prefer the idea of giving birth naturally in a birthing pool with candles, soft music and nothing more than some homeopathic remedies for pain relief.

Although you will always remember your baby's birth, it will fade into the background of your experience once you are a parent. What matters is giving birth to a healthy baby, rather than the exact detail of how the birth occurred.

Hospital birth

Most babies are born in hospital, where they are generally delivered by midwives unless there are complications. The advantage of giving birth in hospital is that there is specialist equipment and care at hand should you need it. If, for example, an epidural is going to be your preferred form of pain relief, then you will need to be in hospital.

Once you've actually had your baby, you may be keen to get back home, as a hospital is not the most restful place to spend the first days with your newborn. It can be reassuring to have care at hand when you don't feel confident about looking after your newborn baby, but maternity wards are often busy and noisy. Most women who have had a straightforward delivery will be out of hospital within 48 hours, and you may not even need to stay that long.

Maternity unit

If you don't like the idea of having your baby in hospital, an alternative is a midwife-led maternity unit. Some maternity units are based in hospitals and others are in the community, but they offer a more relaxed atmosphere than a traditional hospital unit which would be led by a consultant. Some of these units can offer complementary therapies to help you during the birth, and birthing pools if you'd like a water birth. If you've had difficulty getting pregnant, that in itself doesn't rule out the option of a maternity unit, but some won't take women who are above a certain age, or those who are considered to have a greater risk of a complicated delivery. If there are problems during the birth, or if an epidural or a Caesarean is needed, women have to be transferred to a consultant-led unit.

Independent birthing centre

There are also some private maternity units, or birthing centres, which work in a similar way to the state maternity units. They can be extremely expensive, but in return they may offer a high level of individual attention and calm and peaceful surroundings, with birthing pools and complementary therapies often included in the package; however, there is always still a possibility that you might need to transfer to a hospital if there are any complications.

Who does what?

When you are pregnant, there are a number of different people who may help care for you during the pregnancy and birth. Here are some of the main people you may meet:

The obstetrician

An obstetrician is a doctor who specialises in caring for women during pregnancy and birth. They tend to focus on women who have more complicated pregnancies and they get involved in the labour if there are difficulties.

The midwife

Generally, a midwife can provide all the care necessary for a woman during pregnancy and labour. She will refer on to the obstetrician if necessary.

Anaesthetists

Although midwives are trained to offer some forms of pain relief, such as entonox – a pain-relieving gas which is a mixture of oxygen and nitrous oxide – they cannot administer more sophisticated anaesthesia. If you are going to have an epidural – a very effective form of anaesthetic, which is injected into the spine – this will have to be administered by a trained anaesthetist.

Independent midwife

If you want to be sure you know the midwife who will be with you throughout the pregnancy and birth, then you can opt to pay for an independent midwife. Most independent midwives look after women who have chosen to have home births, but some work with hospitals too, and they would be able to remain with you if you had to transfer to hospital. Having an independent midwife ensures continuity of care, but it isn't a cheap option.

Doulas

A doula is someone who comes along with you to the birth to offer support. A doula is not medically qualified, but will focus just on your needs during birth. This can be really helpful, especially if you don't think your partner is going to deal with birth very well! A doula plays the role of an experienced friend who is there just for you, and this is great if you are feeling insecure or anxious about the birth. You would have to pay for a doula, but it doesn't cost nearly as much as a private birthing centre or an independent midwife.

Going to hospital

One of the things that often worries women before they have a baby is how they will know when labour starts.

This can be another of those areas where women who have taken a while to get pregnant start to worry that they will not be sufficiently in tune with their bodies to be certain whether they are really having contractions. There may be weeks, or even months, of occasional weak contractions (known as Braxton Hicks contractions), which help the uterus get ready for the real ones that occur in labour. There may also be false contractions leading up to the birth, which can make you think that labour has started.

Don't feel embarrassed if you end up dashing to hospital only to be told that you aren't yet in labour. Many women experience false labour and it can come and go for a while before the real labour begins. It doesn't mean that you are in any way less capable if you think you are in labour when you aren't – it's just a sign that your body is preparing itself, and shows that things are getting underway.

Induction

If your baby is more than a fortnight overdue, or there are reasons to believe that there are any problems developing, the medical team may decide to induce labour. Sometimes older women, those over 40, are told that induction at term is necessary to 'avoid complications'. If you don't have any objections and would prefer to get things underway, that's fine, but if you would rather wait, you don't have to agree to induction right away and can always ask for a few days' grace to see whether the baby arrives naturally.

There are a number of methods used to induce labour

and you may be given pessaries, your waters may be broken artificially and you may be given oxytocin, which will stimulate labour. Apparently, induction is sometimes suggested for women who are expecting an IVF baby purely because it is considered to be a 'precious baby', but this is something you should discuss carefully with your midwife and doctor if there are no other reasons for inducing your baby and make sure that you feel happy about this before going ahead.

Caesarean section

It is not uncommon for women who've had trouble conceiving to decide that they want to have a Caesarean section, because they feel that this may be the safest way to deliver a long-awaited baby. In fact, there is no reason for your birth to be any more risky just because it took you a while to get pregnant, unless there are other factors that come into play. Having a baby after fertility treatment is not in itself an indication of the need for a Caesarean; however, if you feel that having weighed up all the odds you really would prefer to plan to have a Caesarean in advance, you are likely to get a more sympathetic hearing than someone who conceived without any difficulty.

The medical factors which would normally lead doctors to recommend a planned, or elective, Caesarean are actually fairly limited. You would usually only be offered a planned operation if your baby is in a breech position, which means he would come out bottom first, or if you have placenta praevia (a condition when the placenta is covering part of the entrance to the womb), severe pre-eclampsia (pregnancy-related high blood pressure), a viral infection such as HIV or hepatitis C, an unusually small birth canal or any other medical condition that could make a normal delivery risky.

Caesarean sections are so common, with a quarter of all babies in the UK being delivered this way, that we tend to think of them as being a fairly minor procedure, but a Caesarean is a major abdominal operation. With any such operation, there is always a risk of infection, and it will take about six weeks to heal and fully recover. This is far longer than it would normally take a woman to get back to normal after a vaginal delivery, and you should take this into consideration when you are making your decisions.

More often than not, women who have a Caesarean haven't planned to do so beforehand. If there are complications during labour, an emergency Caesarean will often be carried out. This can happen if the labour is progressing very slowly, if the baby is not getting enough oxygen or if there is any kind of emergency that means that the baby needs to be delivered quickly. In women who are over 35 it often takes longer for the cervix to dilate, or open, and a Caesarean may be necessary if labour is taking too long. Having an emergency Caesarean can be quite a traumatic experience, but sometimes if it comes at the end of a difficult labour it can be more of a relief.

The expert view

Professor James Walker, Royal College of Obstetricians and Gynaecologists

'Caesarean section is directly associated with age. It's not just because you are an older woman and therefore people are leaping in more often, there seems to be a factor related to age which relates to the efficacy of labour itself and which increases the chances of having a section. If you have someone who wants a Caesarean section then it is quite difficult to argue against it on safety grounds. If you've got an IVF pregnancy and you are 38 and you say this is my only one and very precious pregnancy, then an elective section is quite a reasonable thing to opt for; however, if someone wants more than one child, we would strongly argue for a vaginal delivery, because if you've had a previous section, that increases your risk in the next pregnancy. So you are increasing the overall risk by having a section the first time, and what you gain in the first pregnancy, you more than lose in the second pregnancy.'

Naomi's story

Naomi and her partner, Ben, had their baby after their first cycle of IVF, and had been planning a natural birth.

'The birth was not what I had hoped for. I went into labour at two o'clock in the morning when my waters broke. I jumped out of bed and my husband put the light on, and there was loads of blood in my water. We phoned the hospital and they said we needed to go in right away and we had to call a taxi or otherwise they would send an ambulance. I ended up having a Caesarean, and part of the reason I had it was because I told them that I'd been through IVF. They were saying what they'd normally do was induce me and then give me an epidural because of the unexplained bleeding, which could be the placenta detaching, which could be a danger to the baby. I said it sounded really unpredictable and I had been through fertility treatment and it was probably the only child I was ever going to have. I just really didn't want any sort of risk and so they said that in that case I could have a Caesarean, so that's what I ended up having, which was pretty unpleasant but at least he got here safely with the minimum of trauma.

'I had put a lot of pressure on myself to have a natural birth. I did loads of active birth classes and yoga and hypno-birthing. I think I was putting a lot of pressure on myself to have a natural birth because I hadn't had a natural conception and it was really important to me. By having a Caesarean, I felt as if I had failed in some way, and that I had failed at both ends of the process. I'd needed medical intervention to achieve what other women just did completely naturally. It can be a bit of a blow to the ego if you let it.

'As time has gone by I've let those feelings go and in some ways I feel lucky that I had the birth I did. The further away from the birth you get, the less important it is. It just becomes part of your story and you accept it, like you accept that you needed IVF.

'The first time I saw him, they held him up above the blue sheet and he was purple and screaming. I was really frightened by the operation, the only other time I'd been in a similar situation was during the IVF – and so for the 45 minutes when they were sewing me up, my husband was holding him just right by my head. I could see him but I was shaking and my whole body was convulsing. I just couldn't stop shaking and I couldn't engage with him – it was a bit weird.

'When they took me through to recovery, my husband asked if I wanted to try feeding him and he unwrapped him and put him down on me so we could have some skin-to-skin contact. I was lying down and he was just like a bird the way he almost flew down onto me and he just latched on straight away and started feeding. I had the biggest rush of oxytocin that I have ever experienced in my entire life. I was on this incredible high – it was amazing, absolutely amazing, and that for me is the moment when I met him.

'When I was waiting for them to get the operating theatre ready for me I was chatting to the midwife about IVF. I said that dealing with infertility had been the most challenging experience of my life. She laughed and said, "That's because you haven't had children yet!" As the weeks have passed and I have settled into motherhood I've realised I don't agree with her. Yes, being a mum is incredibly challenging, in ways I never expected. But it's nothing compared to managing the pain of infertility for the rest of your life.'

Home birth

Although it is relatively unusual, some women who've had fertility treatment decide that they would like a home birth. The idea of a low-tech natural birth after such a high-tech conception can seem tempting, but do your research first and be aware that you may need to revise your plans at a later date. Not everyone who plans to have a home birth will end up having their baby at home, and it is important to be realistic about this.

There are undoubtedly many merits to having a home birth, but there are also some risks and disadvantages and it is important to be thoroughly aware of them all before you make your decision. One of the major risks with a home birth is that if things get complicated, you may need to be moved to hospital, and it's the moving from one place to another during labour that can be particularly problematic.

I had my first IVF baby in hospital, but my second was a planned home birth. There were, however, circumstances which made that seem a viable prospect. With our first baby, we had been fortunate to come under the care of an amazing group of community midwives who offered caseload midwifery, which meant that the same two midwives cared for you throughout pregnancy and during the birth itself. When I got pregnant for the second time, I was able to access the same care and the same two midwives. By this time, I counted them both as friends and trusted them implicitly. Having a home birth in the hands of two trusted and experienced midwives who I knew well and who had been with me throughout two pregnancies didn't feel risky. We had the added bonus of living just minutes away from our local hospital, but everything went well and my daughter was born at home. Having spent time with fertility consultants and obstetricians since, I must confess that I've stopped admitting I had an IVF baby at home, as most are so completely horrified and utterly aghast that I could have chosen to take what they see as a great risk for my baby and myself.

So, a home birth doesn't have to be ruled out just because you are expecting an IVF baby, but if you are an older mother or have any other reasons to suspect that labour may be more complicated, it is important to be realistic about this and to weigh up the pros and cons.

The expert view

Professor James Walker, Royal College of Obstetricians and Gynaecologists

'Most problems in labour are not to do with the place of delivery, it's not the risk of you delivering at home, it's the risk of you having to be transferred out and that's the main problem. As for having the first baby at home, remember that home birth in the first pregnancy just doesn't happen in a lot of cases, 40 per cent will be transferred in labour into hospital to have their baby and you've got the added complication of the risk of transfer. If you are 30–40, then 75 per cent of women will be transferred in because of complications. If you have an IVF pregnancy at the age of 38, it's not just the IVF, it's all the other things that go along with it. I am not going to say that you can't have a home birth, what I am going to say is that it is unlikely that you will have a home birth because it is unlikely that you will be successful – complications relating to poor progression in labour and to fetal distress are far more likely to occur in a woman who is 38 than in a woman who is 21.'

Premature birth

Babies are more likely to be premature if they are born after fertility treatment, as some of the factors which are linked with prematurity, particularly multiple pregnancy, are more common after treatment. Care for premature babies has improved hugely over the years, and babies can survive if they are born as early as 22 or 23 weeks, although they will need a lot of help and support.

Any baby born before 37 weeks is classified as being premature, but babies develop very rapidly in the last trimester of pregnancy and a baby born after 34 weeks is generally fairly well developed and so less likely to have breathing problems, which are often a major concern for premature babies. A premature baby usually needs medical care, either in a special care baby unit or in neonatal intensive care, and they may need to be in an incubator at first to ensure they keep warm.

If you go into labour before 28 weeks, you will usually be taken to a hospital which has a neonatal intensive care unit to have your baby. Your baby is likely to need to spend some time on a ventilator at first to help her breathe, as her lungs will not be fully developed. There can be many complications when babies are born this early, and if you've waited a long time to have your baby, it can seem terrifying if you have a very premature birth and a baby who is tiny and weak. You will feel anxious and worried, but make sure you talk to the staff about your concerns so that they can explain what is happening and why. It is difficult if your baby is in an incubator and you may feel that you can't do anything useful, but just sitting and talking to your baby will help you bond. Breast milk is particularly important for premature babies, as it contains antibodies which can help fight against infection, as well as being easier for your baby to digest. If your baby is very small and cannot breastfeed, she can still have expressed breast milk fed through a special tube. Try to remind yourself that your baby is getting expert care from professionals who are experienced at looking after premature babies and know how to give them the special attention that they need. Special care has improved hugely in recent years, and it's not just survival rates that have improved for premature babies but also the long-term prognosis.

Lucy's story

Lucy and Matthew had four IVF cycles, two of which resulted in miscarriage, before Lucy finally got pregnant again.

'When I got to 31 weeks, we went on holiday on a canal boat with some friends and my waters broke at about two o'clock in the morning. We rang the midwife and she said to ring an ambulance. Luckily, we were moored near a lock and the ambulance came and we went into hospital. They said that the head was engaged and that I was in labour. They gave me some steroids but the labour progressed too quickly for them to take effect on the baby's lungs. You imagine this moment where they put the baby on your chest, but I didn't have any of that. They just whisked him straight away and I didn't even see him, but luckily he was alive.

'It was all a bit of a shock. He was in intensive care for

a week and they had to ventilate him, which took 24 hours and was really scary because he couldn't breathe for himself. He was so tiny that we couldn't hold him for three or four days and then they only let me hold him for about a minute. I was feeling as if the whole experience had been taken away – at that point obviously we were just desperate for him to be all right. Initially, I had a huge hormonal euphoria after giving birth even though it was all really traumatic, but then I came crashing down with the reality of the seriousness of it all.

'Then he was moved to a local hospital and we were feeling optimistic that he would be at home in a few weeks, but they couldn't really get to the bottom of what was going on. He just wasn't breathing as he should – his oxygen levels kept going down and his alarm would go off sometimes several times in half an hour. They would all rush in and grab oxygen, and that would happen all the time. They kept disagreeing with each other about what was wrong with him. In the end they gave up and said he had to go to a bigger unit. We were optimistic because it was a newer hospital with better doctors, but then they went round in circles too. When I was trying to give him bottles, he kept choking and they couldn't work out if it was severe reflux or if his airways were constricted. Then he got pneumonia because milk had gone into his lungs and he suddenly went downhill and was moved into intensive care. That was at about eight weeks and he was in intensive care for a week.

'He was three months old when he first came home. He was quite fragile and we were nervous but we got into the swing of it quite quickly. I think the angst has gone.

While he was in hospital I was worried about his bond to me, as he was completely taken care of by the nurses and I wasn't allowed to feed him when I wanted to. It was quite odd.

'I remember the intensity of feeling when he first came home. I don't know if I love him more than any other mother loves her child, but there is an intensity about it. I was so happy from the minute he was born, even when he was so unwell, the love was there from the start, and I feel the most unbelievable joy, happiness and relief that I had a baby in the end after all the ups and downs. He was worth every minute of the heartache and every penny we spent for IVF. At times I feel so lucky, as he is in our lives against the odds – he is a bit of a miracle baby.'

The first sight of your baby

Whatever kind of labour you have, the moment that you will always remember is seeing this tiny person you've been carrying for nine months for the first time. It is an overwhelming experience for both parents, and the trials of labour are often instantly forgotten as you focus on your baby. When you've anticipated this joyous moment for so long, you have probably imagined you would immediately bond with your baby, but although many people do feel an instant and enormous rush of love for their child, not everyone does. There's a greater danger that this moment won't quite live up to expectations when you've waited for it for years. You will probably be exhausted and slightly shell-shocked from labour, and this can leave you feeling numb. This is more common after a particularly difficult labour. Don't worry if you don't feel the sense of closeness and bonding with your baby that you had anticipated right away. It isn't something that has to happen immediately, it is often a gradual process of building a close attachment.

Newborn babies aren't always particularly attractive, as they are wrinkly and often slightly squashed after travelling through the birth canal. They may be covered in downy hair or a greasy, white substance called vernix and their heads are often pointy. I remember very clearly the first sight of my son, all red and wrinkly and smeared with blood. He looked more like a grumpy old man than a small baby. He had taken a long time to be born, and appeared to be extremely cross about the whole experience. To me, he looked perfect, but when you've spent the last nine months imagining some gorgeous rosy-cheeked child, the reality of your own newborn can come as rather a shock.

The midwife will cut the baby's umbilical cord, and check his general condition to make sure that everything is all right. The baby's pulse, breathing, movements, skin colour and reflexes are all measured within minutes of the birth, and again a few minutes later to ensure that there aren't any problems.

Newborn babies often seem terribly fragile, and you may feel anxious about picking your baby up. Most people don't instinctively know how to handle a tiny baby, and if you feel cautious, this isn't some unique failing of women who have found it hard to get pregnant and you aren't lacking in natural maternal responses. Having a child is a huge learning process and most people's first steps on the path are rather hesitant and uncertain.

Kelly's story

Kelly and her husband, Terry, had been trying to have a child for six years. They were overjoyed when Kelly discovered she was pregnant after their second attempt at ICSI.

'My mum said I was mad, but actually I really enjoyed the birth. I had to be induced because my waters broke. I went to the clinic because I wasn't sure it was my waters, and they said it was the forewaters and there was still water round the baby, but if nothing happened within the next couple of days, they would induce me. I went back and they scanned me again and I was getting quite worried that something was going to happen. The lady looked at my papers and she said, "You've had a rough time trying to get this baby haven't you?" And I just broke down, so she said they would bring me in to be induced.

'I am quite a wimp and I didn't think I'd be able to cope with it but I actually surprised myself. I felt fine – I only had gas and air. I was just so excited about actually having a baby that the excitement overwhelmed everything else, and nothing fazed me. They say it is normally more painful when you are induced, but I wasn't really in that much pain. I remember bits that were really painful and I had the gas and air to stop the pain, but it wasn't as if it was so painful that I couldn't control it or that it was overtaking me. I never felt anything like that.

'He was born at nine o'clock the next morning so I was only in labour for seven hours. He wouldn't actually come out so I had to have a ventouse. I was absolutely fine, but my mum said it was horrendous – she was there with my husband. I had been really frightened about the birth – I suppose most people are when it is their first time – I thought it was going to be really bad and it just wasn't. I said afterwards that I wouldn't mind doing it again and my mum just didn't believe it. She's had six children and she said my birth was horrendous, but it was strange, I didn't feel like that.

'I stayed in hospital the first night and I didn't sleep the whole time. I hadn't slept for about two days because I just kept looking at him – I thought if I took my eyes off him he might disappear, so I was just staring at him the whole night while I was in hospital. It wasn't until the next day when I came home and he was with my husband that I fell asleep. I was breastfeeding and it was harder than I had expected for the first week, but then he really latched on and he was just the perfect baby. Silly things can make me cry at the drop of a hat if they remind me of how I felt then – I am never going to feel like that again because I have got my little boy now, but I can still remember how it was.'

CHAPTER 5
The Early Days

One of the most overwhelming times for any new parent is when you bring your new baby home for the first time. No matter how long it has taken you to conceive, or how you have done it, the responsibility you feel for this tiny person is enormous. We imagine that becoming a parent should be the most natural, instinctive thing in the world, but for most people it feels completely daunting. It is quite normal to question whether you really have the skills to care for your new baby who seems so small and vulnerable. Some people appear to take it all in their stride relatively easily, but most of us worry about every sigh, gurgle or snuffle. You may feel anxious when you touch your baby or pick her up because she seems so fragile, but remember that babies are much stronger than you might expect.

Newborn babies often look odd, and not remotely like the picture-book child you may have envisaged when you were longing for a family. They can get spots within the first few days, their skin is wrinkled, their heads may be an odd shape and they sometimes look quite battered after the birth. Their breathing can be irregular and they may make odd noises. It is sometimes hard to establish a bond with your baby right away if all you can see is the strangeness of a newborn, so do remember to allow time for this to happen, as bonding is a gradual process.

Of course, some parents just look at their wrinkly little babies and see a vision of loveliness. I remember being genuinely shocked when an acquaintance, seeing my son for the first time, made a jokey comment about all babies being ugly. I really didn't understand what on earth he was talking about, as to me my baby was utterly delightful. Looking back at photos of his rather cross, scrunched-up face, I can now appreciate that although they still look gorgeous to me, this is perhaps an example of beauty being in the eye of the beholder.

When it isn't what you'd expected

When I brought my son home for the first time at just a few hours old, I found it hard to believe that I was going to be left with this tiny creature without constant professional help, as I felt that I didn't have a clue how to look after him. It was like being handed some hugely complex and very delicate piece of equipment without a manual. It was overwhelming at first, but once you get used to it, a baby's needs are fairly simple – initially all they want to do is feed, sleep and have their nappies changed. What *is* a complete mystery is the way that such simple needs can take up every single moment of your day.

If it has taken you a while to get pregnant, you may

have started avoiding other people's children and babies.
I got to a point where I wouldn't even hold babies and I
sometimes felt other people must imagine my apparent
total lack of any maternal instinct might be in some way
responsible for my fertility problems. The truth was that
I couldn't bear the pain of holding other people's children,
and was always worried that I might burst into tears. If
you've found it difficult to be around babies and small
children, this can leave you feeling even less able when
you are first left alone with your own baby, as you may
not have spent time with your friends or relatives watching
what they did when they had their children.

Don't worry if you feel that you aren't doing things
properly. In truth, no new parent quite knows what they
are doing at first, and everyone feels as if they have been
thrown in at the deep end. Being a new parent comes
with a really steep learning curve. One of the problems
for parents who have longed for a family for many years
is that you often have completely unrealistic expectations
of the ideal sort of parent you will become, and you want
to do everything perfectly, with no margin for error or
learning. You may have imagined yourself drifting around
with a well-fed dozy baby gurgling happily in your arms,
a row of gleaming white babygros flapping on the washing
line, a tidy, polished house and a healthy supper cooking
in the oven. Finding yourself in your dressing gown at
lunchtime, hair awry, still not having managed to eat
breakfast as you desperately rock a screaming baby is not
the way that you have imagined your family life, and yet
it is probably a far more realistic picture of life with a
newborn baby.

It is really hard work having a new baby, and no one can ever explain beforehand how such a small person can take up so much time and energy. If you start out with very high expectations of how you will deal with parenthood, then you may feel you are failing if you never have time to clean the house, if piles of washing are mounting up and you are always running out of teabags. Try not to worry about domestic chores too much at the beginning. No one is going to judge you for not having done the washing up or the ironing. If you are very houseproud it can be difficult to accept that you may have to let things slide a little, and even for people (like me) who have a more relaxed attitude to housework, it isn't always comfortable to live in chaos. It will get easier and you will have more time once you are used to your baby. What matters now is the time you spend getting to know your baby, not the cleaning and dusting.

With both my children, I felt an odd pressure to get up and out and about as soon as I physically could. I went on a long walk around the park just a few days after my son was born, and wondered why I suddenly felt exhausted and had to collapse on a park bench; photographs of my daughter's early days show me looking really quite unwell as I pushed myself against all my body's natural instincts to start rushing about. In retrospect, I can't imagine why I wanted to get on with things I could have done on every normal day of my life so soon after having my babies. It really doesn't matter if you spend the first week in your pyjamas, and in fact it might be a good idea, as it will ensure that you have some relaxing time with your baby. If your partner has some time off work, this is such a special time for all three of you, and it's absolutely fine if you don't do anything other than enjoy it.

It's a good idea to allow yourself some space for the first month or so. Of course, everyone wants to come and see the baby, but if you aren't careful you can find that you end up exhausted after spending days on end making cups of tea for dozens of visitors, and don't have any quiet time with your baby. You may want to try to limit visitors at first, or just have people over at certain times of the day so that you know you will get some peace and quiet.

Am I cut out to be a parent?

Most new parents feel incompetent now and then, but for those who've taken a while to get pregnant there can be a feeling that everyone else knows something that you don't when it comes to looking after a baby. You may have always assumed that once you had a baby, you would automatically feel just like any other parent and yet somehow you don't. It can be hard to pin down exactly why you still feel different, but you may worry that you are more anxious about your baby, that you find it harder to be separated from him and that you don't feel as confident about your parenting abilities.

At first it is hard to interpret what your baby is feeling, to know when he is tired or hungry. You may feel ill at ease, and it is sometimes tempting to start blaming your-self. When I found things difficult, I would find myself wondering whether my infertility had been a sign that I wasn't cut out to be a parent. When my first baby was just a few months old, we went away for a weekend with friends who all had older children. Their children were tucked up in bed and fast asleep while I was taking ages feeding my son and then trying to settle him. I immedi-ately felt I was failing to become the efficient sort of mother that my friends had turned into, and saw this as a sign of my ineptitude as a parent. I didn't stop to think that a tiny baby and a group of small children are hardly comparable, or that most of my friends would have been doing exactly the same thing with their own babies in the first few months.

We're often too hard on ourselves, and assume that everyone else is doing a better job than we are because they were meant to be parents and we've somehow sneaked into parenthood through the back door. Research shows that people who've been through fertility problems make very dedicated parents and do a better-than-average job despite the fact that we may start out feeling more anxious about what we're doing. If anything, having a fertility problem is likely to make you a better parent rather than a worse one, so keep that in mind if you are worrying about your abilities.

The expert view

Professor Susan Golombok, director, Centre for Family Research, University of Cambridge

'There is some evidence that there are raised levels of anxiety for people who have experienced fertility problems in the first year or so after the birth. Often IVF parents worry because they've been through so much to have a child that they set very high parenting standards and they worry about the child being more vulnerable in some way. That seems to tail off quite quickly and in our studies we find that as the children grow into toddlerhood and beyond, the parents are very involved with their children, very committed to their children and generally the families seem to be doing very well.'

Anxiety about your baby

When it has taken you a while to get pregnant, you've had a lot of experience of things going wrong and it can be hard to believe that something is going right for a change. So many of the people I've interviewed have told me that they found it hard to believe that their baby was really there to stay. There is often an underlying worry that somehow your luck can't have changed so totally, that something must go wrong at some point and that often translates into fears that something is going to happen to the baby.

I don't think I put my son down at all during the first few weeks of his life. When I did put him in his cot to sleep, I would turn the baby monitor up as loud as it would go and keep it close to me so that I could hear his every snuffle. I'd still have to keep going back into his room to make sure it was working properly and that he was OK, and would reassure myself that he was breathing by resting my hand on his chest to feel it rise and fall. If he had the tiniest spot on his skin, I would be rolling glasses over him to check that it wasn't a sign of meningitis. I was probably quite neurotic for the first few months, living with a tinge of fear all the time, unable to believe that we had such a wonderful child and that this happiness could possibly last.

Getting out and about

It takes ages to do anything with a baby, and I was mystified at first by the amount of time it took me to get out of the house. No longer could I pull on a coat, pick up my keys and walk out the front door. Now, before leaving there always seemed to be a nappy to change, a quick feed to be given, a changing bag to be prepared, and by the time I thought I was ready to go, there might be another nappy to change and another quick feed to be given. Don't worry if it takes ages to do anything. This is perfectly normal, it does get easier and you will speed up with time!

Dealing with other people

My first baby was almost entirely nocturnal, spending his days sleeping soundly and the nights wide awake and wanting attention. I remember saying to someone when he was a few months old that it would be blissful to sleep for a whole night sometime. 'But you wanted a baby, surely you're grateful?' she retorted. If I'd conceived naturally, no one would have ever questioned my right to admit to feeling exhausted, or to make any kind of judgement about it. When you've wanted a baby for a long time, you may feel that you are expected to find every dirty nappy and every sleepless night a source of great joy. Other people may seem to assume that you pass your days, and nights, in a state of elation. Some of this, it has to be admitted, is probably in your own head. You know how much you longed for a baby, you feel that you should be endlessly grateful and so you imagine that other people must think this too. What can be hard is admitting, even to yourself, that sometimes having a small baby is just utterly exhausting.

This can mean that parents who've waited a while for their baby feel that they have to constantly prove that they are coping well. If you seem to be handling everything with confidence, other people may assume that you don't want, or need, any help. Actually, new mothers need all the help that they can get and there's no shame in admitting this. Don't be too proud to accept offers of assistance, and don't feel it's a sign of not being a good parent if you let other people help out. If a relative or friend asks if they can do anything, ask them to load the dishwasher or hang out the washing. People like to feel useful so they will go away feeling glad that they've helped, and you'll have one less thing to get done.

The other thing you may find is that people are constantly offering advice and suggestions as to how you should care for your baby. It can be handy if you're not sure about something and it's always worth listening to other people's suggestions, but don't feel that you have to follow everything that everyone else tells you, especially as some of it will be completely contradictory. I was always concerned that other people were finding me lacking as a new parent, and I had little faith in my own abilities to get anything right so I'd veer between one way of doing things and another, probably leaving my poor baby totally confused. My first health visitor said I should swaddle my son and she very efficiently wrapped him up in a neat little bundle, which caused him to scream and struggle manically but she was quite adamant that this was what was necessary. I couldn't ever get him into anything resembling her neat bundle and he seemed to hate being packaged up. The health visitor who came the next week, and they really did change weekly, said that there was no need for any swaddling – much to my relief and my son's.

If you're feeling this way, do be reassured that it will get easier, that you will come to feel confident in your own way of doing things. Don't forget that this is your baby and it's up to you how you bring her up.

Getting support

It's not just the practical things you may need help with but also the emotional side of being a new parent. As with infertility, there's nothing like talking to other people who are in the same situation, as it makes you realise that you're not the only one finding certain things difficult. When I had my first baby, my midwives suggested I went along to a group they ran for mothers with newborn babies. At the time, I couldn't think of anything I wanted to do less, but they were quite insistent about it so I did go and, having gone once, went back again every week.

I didn't realise at the time how lonely many people find it when they are at home with a small baby, because I was fortunate enough to have close family living nearby, a few friends who were also on maternity leave from work and a ready-made social life through the midwives' mother and baby group. Once our babies were a few months old, we stopped going to the mother and baby group and instead went to one another's houses or out to cafes for lunch. I discovered that one of the other mothers had an IVF baby and it really helped to make me feel that I had just as much right to be at a mother and baby group as any other woman with a baby. Fourteen years down the line, these women are still friends. I don't see them often, but we keep in touch and I will always be grateful that I had such a supportive network at the start, as it really did make all the difference. It can also help you feel more confident, as you realise that *everyone* is learning as they go along, and that you can all help one another because there is no one 'right' way to do things.

It's important to get this kind of support. You may well start out thinking, in just the way that I did, that you don't need it. Do give it a go if you can, as it's easy to get stuck in the house when you have a small baby, and not to see anyone else or to talk to anyone all day. There's nothing like spending time with another mother who has a baby of the same age to make you realise that everyone has worries and concerns and that everyone finds it difficult sometimes. Sharing this and making new friends can be the fun part of having a small baby if you let it.

While it is important to ensure you don't get isolated by spending all your time alone with your baby at home, it is equally important to ensure you do what feels right for you. Some women with young babies live in a whirl of coffee mornings and baby classes, but you shouldn't feel pressured into packing your day with activities just because that is what other mothers are doing. Not everyone enjoys endless chats over cups of coffee or dashing from one baby group to the next. There's no merit to be found in forcing yourself to attend events that feel uncomfortable, as this is not going to increase your self-confidence and in this, as with most things in life, there is a happy balance to be struck.

The expert view
Dr Karin Hammarberg, University of Melbourne

'I think that when having a baby has involved consider-able effort and the pregnancy is much wanted, family, friends and health-care professionals, and the women

continued

themselves, may assume that mothering will be unprob-
lematic and fulfilling. It may be that mothers who have
conceived with fertility treatment don't ask for help and
support and therefore don't get the help they need, and
they may even have a sense of failure when they encounter
the kinds of difficulties most new mothers experience.

'If you and others expect that life will be just wonderful
when you finally have a child, the realities of caring for
a baby may come as a shock. Some babies cry a lot, are
difficult to feed, soothe and settle and it is important
that the woman herself, her partner, family, friends and
health-care professionals understand that being a new
mother, especially if the baby is unsettled and cries a lot,
can be extremely exhausting and isolating, whether you
conceive spontaneously or with treatment, and that
needing help is universal and normal.'

Breastfeeding

We all know that breast milk is the ideal food for a baby,
containing all the necessary nutrients in an easily digest-
ible form. It also helps protect the baby against infections,
as the mother's antibodies are passed to the baby through
breast milk. Breastfed babies are less likely to get consti-
pated or to become overweight. Breastfeeding is cheaper
and more convenient and is even thought to help reduce
the risk of breast and ovarian cancer. It is also a good
way to build the bond with your baby.

Breastfeeding, however, isn't always easy. Some women, and some babies, may take to it instantly without any problems, but most people need some help to establish successful breastfeeding. It can take a while to get the positioning right so that the baby is properly latched on, and some women suffer from very sore nipples when they start feeding. If you experience any difficulties with breastfeeding, do ask for help. It is really common to have problems, whether it's a low milk supply, blocked milk ducts or thrush, and your midwife or health visitor can give you advice. If you need more ongoing help than they have time to give, you should seek out a breastfeeding counsellor or group. Your local branch of the NCT or the La Leche League should be able to help (see Resources).

If you're going to breastfeed successfully, don't forget that you need to look after yourself. Producing sufficient milk for a baby isn't easy unless you are taking time to eat properly, to make sure you are drinking lots of fluids and aren't getting too tired. Sometimes not taking care of yourself properly can cause problems with your milk supply. This is not the time to be thinking about losing any excess weight you have gained during pregnancy either, as you really need to eat well to feed successfully. I ate far more when I was breastfeeding than I ever did when I was pregnant and seemed to have a voracious appetite.

For anyone who has had difficulty getting pregnant, breastfeeding can become hugely significant in terms of what you feel you ought to be able to do as an ideal parent. Current attitudes to breast milk can sometimes leave anyone who is simply unable to breastfeed feeling like an abject failure and a neglectful parent. Of course, in an ideal world you would be breastfeeding your baby, but some women really do find it very difficult. The lack of effective support and guidance can be to blame, but if you've sought out help and are still finding that attempting to breastfeed is making you utterly miserable, don't feel that you would be failing your child if you used formula milk. Every day that you've tried to breastfeed will have helped your baby, but it's far better to have a relaxed, happy mother who is bottle-feeding her baby than an anxious, unhappy, stressed mother who experiences great pain and discomfort every time she attempts to feed her baby. If you and your baby are both happier if you are not constantly struggling unsuccessfully to breastfeed, don't worry about what anyone else thinks.

Routines?

Nothing divides parents, and parenting experts, like the arguments about routines for young babies. On the one hand, we are told that routines are too strict for tiny babies, that they are for selfish parents who put themselves first, on the other that babies will benefit from establishing a regular pattern of sleeping and feeding where their needs are paramount.

I was of the haphazard school of parenting and I am not sure I would have ever been sufficiently organised to establish a regular routine for my children when they were babies. Having come to understand more about routines, however, I can see how incredibly helpful they are to many parents. If you are feeling completely at sea, and this is certainly a common feeling for parents who have taken time to conceive, then having a routine to follow can be a great advantage. There are, of course, some people who find that trying to follow a routine makes them feel more of a failure if they can't get it right, but I suspect a lot of this is down to personality type. If you are an orderly person, then establishing a routine will come to you far more easily than it would for someone of a less efficient and methodical bent. The exception to this rule is parents who have twins and triplets for whom a routine seems to be pretty much essential whatever their nature.

Being an older mother

Looking after a small baby is utterly exhausting, and this level of exhaustion can be harder to cope with if you are an older mother. Most women who've had fertility problems are certainly older than they would have liked to have been when they have their first baby, and you may find yourself regretting this when you see younger mothers dashing effortlessly about with their babies. Although the tiredness may affect you more if you are older, at the same time you may find that you are better equipped to deal with it and more willing to accept the limitations that life with a small baby requires.

Having a child after a long period of fertility problems can make you feel slightly outside the loop with other mothers when you first have your baby, and being an older mother can exacerbate this if all the other new mothers around you seem to be in their twenties while you are in your forties; however, women are having their first babies later now, including those who don't have fertility problems, and there are far more 40-something mothers out there. Talking to other older mothers can be helpful, and you can always do this online if everyone else with a newborn in your area seems to be much younger.

The expert view
Lindsey Harris, Mothers 35 Plus
(www.mothers35plus.co.uk)

'There are some possible health issues for older mothers and you may feel more tired, but there are definite advantages too. Women often feel more settled and more ready in themselves, possibly due to already having had a career and leisure opportunities. They may be more willing than their younger counterparts to make the necessary sacrifices that having a baby inevitably means. They're possibly better able to cope with the emotional and the financial aspects too. And what's more, it can keep you young at heart.'

Looking after yourself

Mothers are notoriously bad at making time for themselves, and mothers who haven't got pregnant easily are probably worse than most others. It's surprisingly easy to forget to eat properly when you are looking after a small baby, and you may find it hard to get outside the house and get some fresh air or to spend some time with other people. Other new mothers are good people to hang out with as they will understand if you are so tired that you can't talk straight and have stains on your jumper, and they won't expect to come round to a pristine house and homemade biscuits. It's so easy to get completely consumed by looking after your baby, but in order to do this effectively you need to take care of yourself as well. If your partner is at work all day, do get him to care for the baby for a while during the evening and, instead of putting a load of washing on, relax in the bath for half an hour with a good book, or even have a quick nap. Do try to remember to snatch some me-time when you can, as this will help you care for your baby more effectively.

Don't worry – and try to enjoy this time!

The early days at home with your new baby are a very special time, but they can be far more difficult than you would ever have anticipated. It feels quite strange and almost alien at first, everything is so complicated and there are so many new issues to worry about. No matter how many baby books you've read or how many people you've talked to, there's really nothing that can prepare you for the enormous impact a new baby has on every area of your life. You may feel that you don't have the skills to look after your baby, or that you can't possibly be doing things properly because you haven't managed to do any housework for a week. Try to remember that it's not because you waited so long for this that it feels so overwhelming, it's like that for everyone regardless of how they conceived their newborn baby.

Naomi's story

Naomi and Ben had two rounds of treatment with Clomid before they tried IVF and were successful first time. When we spoke, their son was two and a half months old.

'I was pretty anxious in the weeks leading up to the 12-week scan, but I was really determined to enjoy it because I felt as if I had been through such a lot to get to that point that I just really wanted to enjoy the experience. There is nothing that divides women like whether or not you've got children. I do feel as if I am in a different world now, and it is quite bizarre having been on the other side for so long.

'Our son is ten weeks now and the last ten weeks have been a bit of a dream. It has been very intense, very over-whelming and I just can't believe he is real after years and years of yearning for a baby and feeling as if I was grasping at air. Having a baby that is mine and that no one is going to take away from me – it's just been absolutely completely and utterly overwhelming. I'm really quite euphoric.

'I've had moments of feeling tired, but I think it has been tempered by knowing that the pain of infertility is far, far worse than anything that I am feeling. In order to go through IVF, I let go of a lot of the ambiguities around having children in order to get through the process. I am so aware that I have friends who are either going through fertility treatment or have been told that they are never going to be able to have children and I know that what they are going through is so much more painful than any sort of tiredness or whatever I might experience. I am possibly not allowing myself to feel any negative feelings because I know I am so unbelievably lucky. It has made me genuinely deeply appreciative of every single moment, and I have to say I feel as if I am living in every moment much more than I normally do. Having a baby demands you to be really present and in the moment anyway because you are just responding to their needs, but I am taking a lot of joy and delight in it too. It's like the joy I feel is the inverse of the depth of pain that I experienced last year, and it is exactly what I imagined it would be. It is possibly even better.

'I felt quite anxious after the birth, and that anxiety hasn't gone. I wasn't prepared for that kind of low-level anxiety that is there constantly – people say that's just being a parent. Because I'd had a Caesarean there was less that I could do, I was having to lie down and it wasn't how I'd imagined the first few days. It was magical the three of us together – it was definitely a kind of baby-moon feeling. In some ways it feels really real now, but on other days we just kind of stare at each other and say, "We've got a baby, we're a mum and dad."

'One of the biggest issues for me has been to what extent you disclose how you got pregnant, and I have not really told many people. When I was pregnant I felt very different, I didn't feel as if I was normal, but once you've got the baby it feels more the same, I feel the same as other women. I think other people may have very different attitudes and may just be completely open about the fact that they'd had IVF, but I felt such a sense of shame that I'd needed IVF – rightly or wrongly – that we'd only told a handful of close friends and family. You are aware of the difference between having sex and just falling pregnant and going through a hugely painful and emotionally draining process – it just separates you out a little bit if you let it. I think I had really felt the stigma of it but now that he is here and he is so gorgeous I have felt it less – I just feel so grateful, my overwhelming feeling is gratitude and I think the feeling of shame is lifting.'

CHAPTER 6

Postnatal Depression

You might imagine that no one would ever experience post-natal depression if they'd been trying for a long time to get pregnant, but in fact it is just as common among women who've had fertility problems and have spent time getting pregnant as it is among the general population. If you've spent years imagining how wonderful it will be if you ever manage to have a baby, the reality of exhaustion, a crying baby and endless nappy changing can be a long way from the rosy image you may have created in your mind.

Many women find it difficult to cope in the early days, and it is extremely common to have what is called the 'baby blues' within the first few days of the birth. You may find that you are very tearful and emotional, and that you experience huge mood swings. This is partly due to the physical and psychological changes you are going through, which involve a huge readjustment in the way you live your life and see yourself. The tearfulness that many women experience in the first six weeks and the feeling that you can't cope will not usually last for long. Generally, the baby blues will gradually disappear as you adjust to life with a small baby. Postnatal depression is a longer-term condition, where the unhappiness persists and the tearfulness doesn't go away. It is a common condition and as many as one in ten women experiences some degree of postnatal depression.

The expert view
Mollie Graneek, specialist fertility counsellor

'Postnatal depression is a very complex disorder and I think it is one that is very often missed. Sometimes it is very hard for women to reconcile with childbirth and babies after IVF. After IVF women feel that they have no right to be depressed, they feel they should be rejoicing in this baby. It just seems like another failure after having to concede to IVF in the first instance and then to say you're feeling a bit depressed – you aren't meant to, you are meant to be happy and grateful.'

How would I know if I had postnatal depression?

Postnatal depression occurs in the first year after your baby is born, and is most common in the first six months. There are some signs which may indicate that you are suffering from postnatal depression.

- You may feel tearful and find that you are crying a lot.

- You may feel overwhelmed by everything and unable to cope.
- You may feel constantly guilty.
- You may find it hard to sleep.
- You may feel exhausted and lacking in energy.
- You may feel tense or irritable.
- You may feel you have lost the ability to enjoy life.
- You may feel very isolated and lonely.
- You may have a poor appetite.
- You may find it hard to concentrate and difficult to make decisions.
- You may blame yourself for everything, feeling that you are not a good mother.
- You may experience panic attacks.

Of course, all new parents feel exhausted, irritable and overwhelmed sometimes, but if this begins to dominate and you are really not enjoying life at all, then it is important to talk to someone about this. If you've had a hard time getting pregnant, the fact that everyone around you is expecting you to be so overjoyed and happy can just add to the pressure that you feel and your sense that you are somehow failing as a mother. We all know how not being able to get pregnant can make you lose self-confidence, and getting pregnant doesn't just automatically reverse this. Your fertility problems may have left you feeling more vulnerable, insecure and full of self-doubt.

Some women are more at risk of postnatal depression, and that includes those who have been depressed in the past. Many women who experience infertility will have had some degree of depression and may have been on what is often described as the emotional roller-coaster of fertility treatment before they ever got pregnant. None of this is easy to deal with, and you will have gone straight from one intense emotional experience into the emotional whirlwind that pregnancy, birth and early parenting can often be.

You're also more likely to experience postnatal depression if you had a difficult pregnancy or if your baby has been unwell or needed special care. Mothers of twins and triplets are more at risk because it is just such hard work to look after more than one baby, and because there are more often health issues with the babies. If you have any family history of postnatal or antenatal depression, that can make a difference too. Sometimes isolation can be a factor, and women who've had fertility treatment may not immediately feel that they are exactly the same as other mothers and able to join in with the mother and baby groups that can offer invaluable postnatal support. If you are dealing with any other stresses in your life, such as financial problems or bereavement, that will increase the risk of postnatal depression too.

Dr Karin Hammarberg has researched postnatal and antenatal depression in women who have had some form of assisted conception. She found that although rates of antenatal depression are far lower than average because the women were so looking forward to becoming parents, their rates of postnatal depression were just the same as those for women who have conceived naturally.

The expert view

Dr Karin Hammarberg, University of Melbourne

'Becoming a mother is an important event in any woman's life; however, when the path to motherhood has been complicated by infertility and infertility treatment, it may be more emotionally complex. It is well known that infertility and infertility treatment are emotionally demanding and that over time these experiences can reduce women's confidence in themselves and their body. Very high expectations of life with a new baby may have left some women a bit unprepared for the extraordinary demands involved in caring for a newborn, and the tiredness and the loneliness that most new mothers experience. This together with a degree of distrust in their own ability to sustain, feed and settle the baby may explain some of the early parenting difficulties the mothers in our study experienced.'

Bonding problems

We know that it can take far longer to bond with your baby than many parents expect. If you were anticipating an overwhelming burst of instant love for your baby and this doesn't happen, you might feel that something is terribly wrong, but it may just be that you had extraordinarily high expectations of how you would feel when you finally saw your child. Try to remember that it takes time to build up a relationship with your baby and that

the bond between you may grow gradually. You will probably find that day by day, you start to feel closer to your
baby and more comfortable with him.

If you feel completely detached from your baby, however,
and don't have any feelings for him at all, and if you find
yourself wondering whether you did the right thing in
having him, or even wishing he wasn't there, then this
suggests that there is a deeper problem. This kind of
attachment difficulty can be triggered by postnatal depression, and you may be more at risk if you had a traumatic
birth or have had other problems. If you feel you are
experiencing bonding problems that aren't improving, then
you should talk to someone about this and get some help
and support by following the guidance below for those
who think they may have postnatal depression.

What should I do if I think I have postnatal depression?

When you are feeling really low, it can be difficult to
believe that you are capable of doing anything about your
situation, but it is vital to get some help. Talk to your
partner, a family member or friend about how you are
feeling, and go and see your midwife, health visitor or
family doctor. Don't feel that you are being a bad parent
if you need help, or that you will be judged. Getting some
assistance is the most important thing you can do, and
it will help you to feel better more quickly.

Sometimes all that is needed is support and advice.
Those around you may not have realised how you have

been feeling, and getting some practical help from friends and family so that you can catch up with yourself and have a little time away from your baby now and then may be all that you need. Sometimes joining a mother and baby group can help, and it may be particularly useful if you can seek out a group for those who've had fertility problems in the past or for new mums who have experienced postnatal depression or bonding problems. You will find some details at the back of the book.

Your doctor may suggest a course of antidepressants to help with some of the symptoms you may have been experiencing. Don't feel that this would be a sign of failure, as antidepressants may be able to help sort out some of the issues that have been causing problems, such as sleeplessness, panic attacks and irritability. Once you're able to get some sleep and to stop feeling so anxious or hopeless all the time, you will find it easier to get on with things, and caring for your baby can start to seem less challenging. There are a number of different types of antidepressant and they can take a few weeks to start working. Usually you will need to take them for a few months at least in order to ensure that your symptoms don't come back as soon as you stop. You can still breastfeed with some types of antidepressant, so talk to your doctor about this.

Other sources of support

If you've had counselling during your fertility treatment and found it helpful, it may be a good idea to talk to a counsellor again now. Some counsellors do specialise in this area, and there are details of counselling organisations at the end of the book. Psychological treatments such as cognitive behaviour therapy can be successful for women with postnatal depression but they do involve a longer-term commitment and may not be as easily available.

There may be things you can do for yourself if you are able to. Looking after yourself is important, so make sure you eat properly, get plenty of rest and try to take some exercise. Don't keep battling on alone if you are offered any practical help by friends or relatives, as this can give you a breathing space which may make all the difference. Techniques such as meditation can be helpful too. Try not to put too much pressure on yourself to do everything perfectly, as it really doesn't matter if the washing-up gets left for a while or the house isn't perfectly tidy; it's far more important that you don't stress yourself out trying to do too much. Think about the things that you used to enjoy, and see if you can find some time for them. Of course, when you are really low you may not feel able to do any of these things, but even just taking one small step towards helping yourself will have a positive influence.

Many women use complementary therapies to help when they have fertility problems, and these may be useful for postnatal depression too. When you go to see a complementary therapist they will have time to talk and to listen, and many therapies are very good for helping people to relax and to feel calmer. This is certainly something you may want to consider and it will also give you some time to focus on yourself.

The expert view

Gerad Kite, acupuncturist

'Being pregnant and having a child is all very challenging. It's a new experience and there are so many things converging at once that even the strongest person can easily get knocked off course. It's simply someone not being able to cope with the change – the physiological change, the change in their relationship with their partner, the way that people see them, the responsibility of being a mother. Acupuncture offers people a way of coming back to a place within themselves where they are well, emotionally stable and can cope with things – it's a great support for coping mechanisms.'

Moving on

It may seem as if you will never be yourself again, but although it may take some time and some patience, you will get better. Try to do what you can to help yourself and talk to people about how you are feeling rather than keeping everything bottled up inside. Don't blame yourself for how you are feeling and remember that you will move on and things will get easier.

Alice's story

Alice and David were delighted when Alice got pregnant after her third cycle of ICSI. During the pregnancy she found

*it hard to believe she would ever have a baby, and she had
a stressful birth.*

'All through the pregnancy I was convinced that the baby
was going to be stillborn. We'd been lucky enough to get
a positive test result, and I didn't think our luck could carry
on. I thought that something would happen to take it away
from us. I didn't have a good birth, and I had problems
breastfeeding. The midwife in the hospital told me that I
had flat nipples, which didn't help my self-esteem. I ended
up expressing a lot, but when he was six weeks old I was
ill and couldn't express anything. I felt as if I'd failed because
it was pushed in your face about the breastfeeding so that
was always there like an underlying thing. Everything got
on top of me.

'At about four months I started getting into the Wii Fit
and was feeling good because I was getting the endorphins.
Then I gradually just couldn't do it physically. It wasn't a
case that I didn't want to, I just couldn't. My biggest problem
was myself. I'd been trying to be superwoman. I do like to
be in control and obviously with a baby you can't be in
control. I didn't want to let things go around the house.
My friend said to me if I do one lot of washing in a day
that is an achievement, but I was trying to do it all and get
it dry and ironed – I was trying to be superwoman.

'I was embarrassed at how I felt because we'd been trying
for four years and had been through three lots of treatment, but why did I not feel happy? We had three lots of
treatment in a year and it was quite a short time to have
all that treatment. I didn't believe that my son would be
born and then all of a sudden he was there. I think the

treatment had a lot to answer for. I felt I wasn't a person any more and I didn't have my own identity.

'I did know I couldn't help how I was. I was being so snappy and my poor husband got it all. I felt like a failure. I felt because of the IVF I should be Supermum and I thought people were looking at me as if I wasn't doing things right. It was complete paranoia. What I do with my son now I always used to do, it's not as if I have treated him any differently, but now I can see that what I was doing was good, and that I am good with him. Before, for some reason, I got it into my head that I was no good. I felt I was being punished for something.

'I kept forcing myself to go out to places because my parents kept saying, "You need to get out every day," and I really didn't want to. I had to drag myself to these places. I had been depressed before, after the first treatment, and my way out then was throwing myself into the gym. I knew I was heading that way and I went to this playgroup one day and one of my friends was saying she'd got postnatal depression and she described it quite openly, and I said that I'd been feeling like that. I went to see the doctor when my son was about five months. I have responded quite well to medication, and the doctor says it is looking good, but I am not going to be off the medication for another few months, so it is a long-term thing. The depression was only ever mild – it wasn't like I was ever going to leave my son or hurt him or anything.

'I thought people would think I was a failure. When I told my mother she said I'd been doing a great job. I don't think that there is any support specifically for people who've had fertility treatment. In my case it was because of the birth and because for five years I couldn't be near pregnant people – it physically hurt me and I felt my heart was being ripped out when I saw families in the park, things that I longed to do, and all I could think was that I might never be able to do them. People can't understand what it's like unless they've been through it.'

CHAPTER 7

Family Life

As time passes, you will find that you settle into family life and start to feel more comfortable in your role as a parent. Some of the anxieties of the early days will begin to fade, and your confidence in your own abilities will grow. Despite this, I think most parents who have taken time to conceive would say that their infertility continues to have an influence, although it may manifest itself in more subtle ways.

There are some common themes that run through the family lives of those who had to struggle to become parents. We are aware of how lucky we are to have our children and we have high expectations of ourselves. We want to be good parents and may find it hard to vent the usual frustrations that any parent will feel. We need to learn to feel confident that we are just as able as anyone else, to appreciate that there is no one 'right' way to bring up children and to allow ourselves to enjoy what we have waited so long to achieve.

Becoming a confident parent

It takes time to become a confident parent, and I am not sure that anyone is ever entirely confident that they always make good parenting decisions. Most parents continue to worry about doing the right thing throughout their children's lives as the demands and challenges change, but most also come to terms with the fact that this is just part of normal family life. If you have found it difficult to get pregnant, you may have an underlying fear that you will also find it more difficult to be a parent and it can sometimes feel as if you haven't taken to it as effortlessly as those who got there more easily.

I think our lack of confidence is caused by our high expectations of ourselves, as we are more prone to worry about the normal ups and downs of family life, and to assume it must be our fault if things don't go entirely according to plan. Try to keep upsets in perspective, and to remember that it would be unusual for a toddler not to have occasional tantrums, that no child is always perfectly behaved and that it is quite normal to sometimes feel so exhausted that you wonder what it would be like to walk out the door and leave the mayhem behind. If you think that you should be feeling permanently happy now you are finally a parent, these everyday hiccups can assume a significance that they don't deserve. Talking to other parents can help you to realise that you aren't the only one struggling with different developmental phases and worrying about whether you ought to be doing things differently.

It's vital to remember that the internal chaos we can all feel as parents is often invisible to other people. When my son was at nursery, another mother once remarked on how cheerful I always seemed to be when I was with him. I was amazed as I was forever berating myself for being grumpy and short-tempered, and I found it hard to believe that she had such a completely different vision of me as a parent. You may worry that you aren't doing things properly, but from the outside you may appear to be competent and in control. Most parents feel inadequate at times, and it would be worrying if we didn't, as we have to learn on the job as we go. Try not to let your fears about your parenting skills spoil your enjoyment of your children, as allowing yourself to feel that joy is probably the best way to gain confidence in your abilities.

Being a superparent

It is common for parents who haven't had their children easily to put a huge amount of pressure on themselves to be far more than an ordinary run-of-the-mill parent. There has been such a long build up to having a child, so many years of dreaming about having a family of your own, that it's easy to create an idealistic image of the sort of parent you would be.

This desire for perfection is exacerbated by society's current obsession with parenting, which affects all mothers and fathers regardless of how long it took them to have their children. It is all too easy to end up feeling a failure if you aren't juggling a rewarding well-paid job with providing delicious home-cooked organic meals, if you don't fit in hours of educational play and family craft activities between shepherding your brilliantly talented children from ballet lessons to music classes. Your child will never eat a ready-meal or visit a fast-food restaurant; you won't ever snap at your child or be grumpy, but instead will be there with a calm smile and caring attitude, doing everything you can to make your child's early years as happy and rewarding as possible.

However much parents do, there is always something more that you could be doing, and it's very easy to compare yourself with other parents and decide that you are lacking. It may help if you try to forget about what you feel you ought to be doing, and stop putting pressure on yourself to try to give your offspring a perfect child-hood. Happy memories are often built on small, simple things that you do together and are certainly not made from hours being escorted from one educational experience to another by a stressed and slightly manic parent.

Expert guidance

A visit to your local bookshop or library will reveal a plethora of books on the skills you will need to bring up your child successfully. What was once left to instinct is now an entire discipline and we worry about our parenting skills and ensuring we are following the right sort of parenting guidelines in a way that previous generations would have found quite alien. There are books on how to have happy children, calm children, successful children, on how to communicate with your children, how to get them to eat, to sleep, to play, to talk. Academics conduct research into parenting practice, while the government produces parenting policies which aim to produce well-functioning families. It's hardly surprising that we sometimes feel anxious about doing the right thing when there is so much contradictory advice.

The expert view

Dr Ellie Lee, director, Centre for Parenting Culture Studies

'Parenting isn't just another word for child rearing, it isn't just a description of what you do if you have got children and are bringing them up – it is a very loaded term which has got a social history associated with it. Parenting has become a highly politicised issue and there has been a very obvious shift in this country towards identifying the relationship between parenting children as the main cause of, and solution to, social problems.'

The idea that our parenting skills, or the lack of them, could be responsible for the social problems of the future is an alarming thought. We find ourselves in the middle of a swing in opinions as a generation who get the blame at both ends of the spectrum: as children, we were responsible if we behaved badly and were duly punished; as adults we are responsible for any bad behaviour our children exhibit, because badly behaved children are now generally considered to be the product of bad parenting.

It's hardly surprising that so many parents are reaching for 'how-to' manuals and anyone who has taken a while to get pregnant may be more eager to seek out advice and support than others. In fact, you are most unlikely to need to be told how to nurture and care for your child as a parent who has longed for a family, but it can be difficult to feel confident in your own abilities in the face of so much advice about what you ought to be doing.

The expert view

Dr Ellie Lee, director, Centre for Parenting Culture Studies

'We are encouraged not to trust ourselves. When you have a child you are going to develop a relationship with another person, so how can that possibly be something that you could read an advice book and know how to do it – it defeats common sense. You have to learn to be a parent, but you can't learn it in the way that you can learn maths or physics – it's like lots of things in life, you have to learn it through experience. It is not a skill set. Your feeling about what is the best thing to do emerges from that process of developing a relationship with your children.'

Being judgemental about other people's parenting skills is the other side of this, and it can appear that some mothers divide themselves into tribal camps about this – the working mums versus the stay-at-home mums, the attachment parents versus the routine parents, the state-school parents versus the independent-school parents. Opinions can become entrenched and there is little attempt to understand one another's points of view, or to allow people to make their own choices in peace without criticism. This highly competitive world can feel really hostile when you come into it from a background of infertility.

Many local schools, nurseries and community centres now offer parenting classes, and these can provide an interesting opportunity to build your confidence, if you recognise the limitations of what such classes can offer. I went to parenting classes at my daughter's nursery, imagining that I might learn some secrets of parenting which had thus far eluded me. The classes were useful, but not in the way I had anticipated. They made me appreciate that everyone gets things wrong sometimes and that it was important for my children to learn that real people didn't drift around in a haze of constantly cheerful well-being but did sometimes get irritable or snappy. I finally accepted that shouting now and again wasn't going to damage my children for life, but would in fact leave them better able to deal with conflict in the world outside our family. I'm not convinced that the aim of the course was to make mothers feel that being grumpy was OK, but it was certainly beneficial for me.

Feeling overprotective

Many parents who have taken time to have their children worry that they might be overprotective, and this can be particularly difficult when you have just one child. It is hard to let go, and to strike the right balance between sensible concern about your child and unnecessary fears. Apparently, many more parents are overprotective of their children now, regardless of how long it took them to conceive, and the phrase 'helicopter parents' was coined to describe those who hover over their children, following their every move and wanting to be involved in everything that they do, sorting out any problems or difficulties. Helicopter parents can become so obsessed with risks and potential dangers that they end up restricting what their child is allowed to do in order to eliminate any possible threat to his safety.

It's easy to give in to helicopter tendencies if it took you a long time to have your family. I think I hovered horribly over my first child when he was young, forever worried that he might fall off climbing frames or walls. Then, of course, I worried that my fears had rubbed off on him as he wasn't particularly physical as a small boy and didn't climb trees or get into scrapes. Despite my fears, this certainly didn't do any long-term damage as he has turned into a sports-obsessed 14-year-old, forever coming home with cuts and bruises from playing football or rugby.

The fact that we are so aware of how precious our children are can make it harder for us to be relaxed about what they do and how they do it, but worrying about being overprotective is not always such a bad thing as it does encourage us to actively think about giving our children some leeway and about getting the balance right.

Growing independence

Watching your child grow older can be a bittersweet experience, as the excitement at each step forwards she takes is tinged with sadness for a phase that has gone forever. The milestones in the early years, from learning to walk to starting school, signal a growing independence. It is far less of an issue if you know that you will probably go through each of these stages with another child in the future than it is if you are pretty certain you will never return to them again.

One of the biggest transitions in your child's early life is starting school, and many a mother sheds a tear on the first day, feeling an acute sense of loss and anxiety. It is natural to worry about how your child will cope without you, and you will stress about all the little things you aren't sure she is capable of doing herself – will she forget to go to the loo if the teacher doesn't remind her, will anyone help her button up her coat at playtime, will someone make sure that she eats at least some of her lunch? It may be reassuring to know that children often take change in their stride in a way that can surprise their parents, and tend to rise to the challenge of growing independence. It can be tempting to constantly question your child about what they've been doing and how things have gone, but it is important to try to give them some space and to allow them to tell you what they want to tell you in their own time. It has taken me 14 years to realise that the fewer questions I ask, the more answers I get!

When our children are little, we are in control of what they do and how they do it. Once they start school, they make their own friends and we don't always know everything about their days. The idea of them having a life of their own at such an early age can feel quite unsettling as a parent. When my son was nearly three, we were out shopping one day when I heard someone shouting his name. A little girl was waving excitedly at him and, as she approached, her father and I looked at one another blankly, neither of us having the least idea how our children knew one another. The girl explained that she was in his class at nursery, and I realised she was someone he'd often talked about. It seemed bizarre to be meeting a friend of his in the street who I didn't know at such an early age, and it brought home to me that he was already gaining an independent life of his own.

When your child is little, you will tend to invite other mothers round who have children of a similar age, but once your child is at school, she will start to have a social life and will spend time at her friends' houses without you. It can feel quite strange to know that someone else will be picking your child up from school and taking her home with them, and that you won't be there to remind her to wipe her nose or to eat her broccoli. The first sleepover with a friend is another big step, and having imagined that you will enjoy a night out, you may well find yourself fretting that she will have a nightmare or wake up in the middle of the night feeling homesick. It does get easier with time, but these early milestones can be difficult at first.

We want to protect our children, but being too involved

in their lives is not always helpful. This is particularly true where their friendships are concerned. You can't organise your child's relationships with other children, or sort out her playground battles. Of course, you would want to step in if there was any question of bullying, but it is important to remember that children need to learn how to resolve disputes, and playground tiffs are part of this learning process. If you are forever intervening in your child's friendships, you may make it harder for her in the long run.

Discipline

It can be tempting to give in easily to a much-loved long-awaited child because having a battle of wills is upsetting for everyone, but setting boundaries and having rules about what is and what is not acceptable, with clear consequences for breaking them, will help your child learn how to behave. You may worry that you are being unkind if you have to lay down the law, but remember that children need boundaries. Those who get away with doing exactly as they please are not usually happy or popular children.

Parents who have waited to have a family are often very concerned about being good parents and are willing to put in the necessary effort to ensure that their children are well brought up. Having a joint policy and sticking to it is essential if this is to work. Of course, no one gets it right all the time, and there will be times when you give in because it's easier, and other times when you find yourself realising that you are adhering to a point of principle which really doesn't matter that much, but we all have our own ideas about what is important. When you talk to other parents you may find that you are comparatively laid back about certain things while being far more strict about others. Try not to worry about what other people are doing, or what they think you ought to be doing, but have confidence in yourself and learn from your mistakes.

'We'd waited so long for Nathan that once he arrived I didn't want anything to go wrong for him. I do worry that sometimes I let him get away with things, but I hate feeling that I am telling him off all the time. Of course, I wouldn't let him do anything really naughty, but to be honest some-times when it's a cheeky little thing I find it quite sweet and I don't want to crush his individuality. There was an occasion recently where he acted a bit spoilt in front of some other parents, and maybe it was me being paranoid, but I did think I could feel their disapproval. I often worry that people are thinking I indulge him because he's an only child but he's a lovely little boy and I know that's what really matters.'
                                                            Elaine

When the going gets tough

Being a parent is hard work, and once you have a child, you often wonder how on earth you filled your life before-hand; what did you do all day and how did you ever feel you were busy? Having someone else take up every moment of your time is exhausting, and you don't become immune to the difficulties of being a parent just because you have wanted a child for so long. It doesn't mean that you will have an amenable, easy child either. Just like adults, children have good and bad days, and being a parent can be demanding.

One common thread for parents who have taken time to conceive is a feeling that they can't ever complain if things get difficult. We know how close we came to a life without children, and this can make it harder to admit that things are not always perfect, that life with young children can be utterly exhausting and that there is a downside to the joy you experience.

In our bid to be perfect blissfully happy parents all day every day, we don't always allow time and space for ourselves either, but this is essential if you want to function properly. Don't feel guilty about needing time away from your children now and again, or about admitting that it can be tough. You will be far more able to face up to the challenges successfully if you have given yourself the space to recharge your batteries and allowed yourself to vent your frustrations.

Going back to work

Most working mothers feel some sense of guilt about leaving their children with someone else during the day, but this can be particularly acute if you have waited to have your child. If you enjoy your work and find it satisfying, going back will be easier, as you won't spend entire days wishing you were at home with your child. It is more difficult if you have to work because you would not be able to survive financially without the income from a job that you don't particularly like. If this is the case, you may want to consider whether you could perhaps work part time or reduce your hours, or even start looking for something that you would find more rewarding.

There is a strange divide between working mothers and stay-at-home mothers, and the intensity of feeling about it can veer towards animosity on both sides. In reality there are advantages and disadvantages to staying at home and to working, and the need to justify a decision that has meant some degree of sacrifice on either side is in part to blame for the schism. For those of us coming from a background of fertility problems, the guilt tripping indulged in by other mothers can strike particularly deep. Mothers who stay at home are often acutely aware of the long-term damage they are causing their future career prospects and may sometimes feel that they have drifted into a backwater of endlessly exhausting domestic duties, losing their identity and status along the way. Mothers who work may feel intensely guilty about leaving their child with someone else all day and worry that this could lead to problems in the future.

'I went back to work full time at the end of my maternity leave. I didn't think about not going back. It wasn't an option financially, and my career is important to me. I tend to work quite long hours so our daughter is at nursery all day. I know it's a long day but I think the social aspect is good for her, as we don't have any friends with kids her age because we are much older parents. Other people are a bit funny about it though, particularly the other mothers at the office who are part time. They often ask me how I can cope with working full time, and are incredibly nosey about our childcare arrangements – I can't imagine what they'd say if they knew she was an IVF baby.'   *Sharon*

Choosing the right childcare

Feeling happy with your childcare arrangements will make all the difference to how you feel about being back at work. There are many types of childcare, and whether you choose a nanny, a day nursery or a child-minder may depend on your working hours, your views about how children should be looked after and your finances. When you are very aware of how precious your child is, you may find it hard to feel confident about leaving him with anyone else at first. You should always trust your instincts and never feel pressured into choosing anything that doesn't feel right. Remember to start looking well in advance and to take time to make a decision. If you know you have made a good choice and if you are confident that your child is happy, it will make things much easier.

Being a stay-at-home mother

When you spend a long time trying to get pregnant, it can start to influence the way you feel about work and a job that has been a central focus in your life can become less appealing. You may even have wondered whether work stress was affecting your fertility and ended up resenting your job. Once you have your child, you may find that you don't have the desire to return to work because you want to savour every possible moment of being a parent.

I went back to work part time after my first baby, but didn't feel quite the same enthusiasm that I'd had before I became a mother. Eventually, when we were trying for a second child, I took a year's unpaid leave and never went back. I was lucky as I didn't ever find it boring being at home with the children, perhaps partly because I always did some freelance work. In the longer term, I am aware that the consequences for my career and earning potential were more devastating than I might have anticipated, but for me that was a price worth paying.

Friendships

Going through infertility can be very testing for friendships. If your friends were all having families while you were still stuck in the maze of fertility tests and treatment, your friendships may have suffered and it can be hard to rebuild relationships that were swept away by the differences in your lives, or even by thoughtless comments or actions. Once you have a family of your own and are in a happier place, it may be easier to forget and forgive.

Sometimes you may feel that other people are judgemental about the lengths that you have gone to in order to have your child, and you may find that you face tactless or unhelpful remarks. This can be particularly difficult if you have used donor eggs or sperm or a surrogate. If some friendships do fall by the wayside, try not to worry unduly, as true friendships will survive and will be able to grow again.

Your relationship

We are all only too aware of the damage that infertility can do to your relationship, and years of baby-making sex to order can leave a legacy. Having a young baby may not make matters any easier. You have little time to yourselves, and birth and breastfeeding don't leave most women feeling particularly sexy. The permanent exhaustion many new parents experience often means that you will snap at one another and you may find yourself worrying whether you will ever feel close again.

During your infertility, you will probably have seen one another in an emotionally raw state and at an all-time low ebb, very vulnerable and exposed, and this can leave cracks in a relationship that take time to mend. There may even be a sense of guilt if the fertility problem wasn't a joint one and this may have left one partner feeling inadequate or the other still nursing some resentment about what they had to go through. If you needed fertility treatment and one of you was rushing faster down this route than the other, you may have a sense of being pushed into something that you weren't entirely sure about, no matter how happy you are with your children. Being a parent may have become more important than your partner to one or both of you; you may feel that you have been left with some kind of tacit power struggle or with one of you stepping back and disassociating yourself from the relationship. If you know that there are underlying issues that are causing real problems, you may want to consider counselling. Couples sometimes feel that they shouldn't need counselling once they've got the baby they longed for, but there should be no shame about getting help to sort out a problem.

We know that not all relationships manage to survive infertility. If you are going to make your relationship work, you need to devote some time and attention to your partner. A mother's close relationship with her baby can leave her partner feeling left out, but what often feels like damage at first can turn into glue after a while if you make an effort to ensure that you share the fun of being parents as well as the sleepless nights and exhaustion, and find some time to be together alone without your child now and again.

'We pushed and pushed because the aim was to have a family and we got our family but there's a bit of wreckage and we are still dealing with the fallout of that now. I don't think fertility treatment brings most people together. Sometimes it isolates you from your partner and exposes weak spots. You have to do the work to find out how to put things back together. If you value your relationship, make time for the two of you to put things back into your relationship because otherwise what you are going to end up with is not what you wanted. What is the point of having put all that effort into having a family if at the end of it you don't tend to the relationship once the children come along? You need to give it more attention and that is hard when you have got children, but you have to make the time to sit down and find each other again.'   *Christopher*

Telling your child

If your child was born as a result of assisted conception, you may have thought about what and when you are going to tell them. This is more of an issue if you've had donor treatment, where it is clear that problems can arise if you don't tell and your child finds out later in life, perhaps by mistake. This is covered in more depth in Chapter 11.

I was quite surprised to discover that many parents don't tell their children, even those who have used their own eggs and sperm for fertility treatment. Maybe some feel it is simply irrelevant, or a private issue for themselves and their partner, and others worry about how they will tell their child. There are also issues about privacy, as young children will not understand any sensitivities you may have about other people knowing that you experienced fertility problems. Sometimes people don't tell their children because they are worried that there is a stigma attached to infertility and that other children may treat them differently or be unkind to them. Although you may feel some stigma yourself, this is most unlikely to affect your child, and fertility treatment is so commonplace nowadays that it tends not to be an issue that causes much interest.

As a family we have always been very open about the

fact that our children were both IVF babies. I've written about it from when the children were very little and have always told people. We don't see it as a source of shame, but are very proud of our children and they know how much we wanted them.

If you are able to talk about it from early on, there will never be a time when you have to sit down and tell your children. If you do need to explain to a young child, it is best to keep it simple. All you need to say is that you had to have help to have them and that a doctor put the egg from mummy and the seed from daddy together. People are sometimes worried that they shouldn't tell their children until they understand what happens in normal conception, but you don't have to get into complicated explanations about it and it doesn't need to involve talking about sex at all.

If you have a child as a result of a frozen embryo transfer, that may appear to be more difficult to explain – it's actually quite a complicated concept for many adults to grasp, let alone children. We used frozen embryos when we conceived our daughter, and she has always known this and just accepted it, really without much interest at all. I think it's an issue that may seem more significant to parents than it does to children!

Aspirations and expectations

We all tend to see our children as unique, wonderful beings, extraordinarily bright, funny and interesting. Of course, your child is very special, but sometimes parents can be terribly disappointed to discover that their budding mathematician turns out to be fairly average with numbers once he gets to school, or that the early reader who learnt his letters at three may not continue to progress with reading at break-neck speed. Try not to fall into the trap of comparing your child with others. He is special regardless of his reading level or his knowledge of the times tables, and it's the confidence that your love and attention give him that will help him to become a happy, successful adult, not his academic achievements.

Sometimes we can be guilty of projecting our own failed aspirations onto our children. If you had always secretly wanted to be a musician, you may have dreamt that your child would be a pianist. If you are lacking in self-confidence, you may have hoped that your child would be very outgoing. It can be hard if you start to see some of your own failings in your child, the things that you'd rather not admit about yourself, as we want them to have all our good points and none of the bad ones. Try not to squeeze your child into being what you think they ought to be, but instead learn to respect and appreciate their own decisions and preferences.

Changes to you

Of course, it's something we will never really be able to tell, but many of us do feel that we aren't quite the same parents that we would have been if we'd had our children easily. Some people continue to carry a residual bitterness, and there may always be uncertain feelings towards people who have children effortlessly that they don't particularly seem to want, but the changes to us as parents don't have to be negative. We may be more empathetic and understanding people, and we have learnt that we should never take our children for granted.

Debbie's story

Debbie and her husband had their first child after their third attempt at IVF, and then continued with treatment in order to try for a second. It took some years of treatment before they were finally successful again, using a donor egg in the Czech Republic.

'I think we are much more aware of how precious our children are. I did three IVFs to have the first one and I was 39 when I conceived. I started treatment properly again when she was two, and had another nine cycles, so 12 altogether. I got pregnant on number 11 and miscarried just before the scan – on my daughter's birthday. Everybody said when I miscarried that it was time to give up because it was our eleventh cycle. We were going to live in Hong Kong, and I was thinking of trying to adopt from China, but then we just decided to try one more time. We decided to go ahead, and at the last minute my husband got a job in London and I got pregnant. I have tried twice since then for a third child. We had some frozen embryos left, so we tried them and then did another fresh one. I've done 14 cycles altogether, 14 two-week waits, 14 pregnancy tests.

'We have had marital problems and I don't know if the treatment contributed to them. Since my daughter was two, I did IVF on average every six months. That's a lot of planning. I think I had this thing in my head that because it had worked, I knew it could work again, so I kept plugging away. I don't work, so I had the time to do the research and we were lucky with the money. I don't know how much we spent – it was a huge amount. My husband was supportive, he said "Let's keep going while we've got the money," but he was rubbish as far as emotional support was concerned. I focused on the cycles and maybe it delayed me seeing what was in front of me. I was putting all my energies into it because you have to be strong to go through it. I wonder whether the treatment was part of what drove us apart as a couple, but we have come out of it OK now.

'In September my little one will be going to school every morning and I will be without her, and then in a year it will be all day. I am aware of that loss in a sense and I will feel very sad but I am starting to get involved in other things. For the first two years, you are cocooned in a strange world wrapped around your children, if you don't work, so my daughter going to school will force me to start doing things for myself.

'My second daughter has such a strong personality that I don't even see any of my husband in her, although it was his sperm – she is so much herself, very quirky and strong willed. I've always been very open and talked to my older daughter all about it, but the other day I asked if it bothered her that her sister had come from the Czech Republic, and she said 'She did?' It was a shock to me, as I had told her all about it, because I believe in telling them, but I am not sure if any of it has gone in. She is beginning to ask questions, so I do make sure I bring it up, but she just rolls her eyes when I talk about donor eggs.

'I've always thought I am not a very good parent, because I am not very strict and I am always questioning myself. Other people seem to have it sussed much better. My older daughter is coming to be a pre-teen now but every day I think, *You are fantastic, you are beautiful, I am so lucky you are here.* People have no idea what you went through, and I think you are more conscious of how precious your children are even if you don't realise it is connected with treatment.'

Lulu's story

Lulu had been unsuccessful with IUI before she and her husband decided to try IVF, and they were successful with their first cycle. To their amazement, Lulu went on to have two more children naturally.

'We were about to go for IVF again when our daughter was about 17 months. I had a bit of bleeding between cycles and my GP sent me for a scan, and they said I had a slight growth but that they would check it out later – it was the pregnancy and they missed it. It took me a while to realise I was pregnant. It was only because I'd gone off certain foods. I was shocked and so was my GP – when I said I thought I was pregnant, he asked if I was sure! It was fantastic to be pregnant naturally but tainted by the fact that it was a really bad pregnancy – I had morning sickness and lost weight, he tried to come early and I was in hospital a couple of times for that, and then I got a pelvic problem which affects your joints, so by 30 weeks I could hardly walk. I was really pleased when my son ended up being born early by Caesarean section.

'So at that point we had a girl and a boy, and my husband

didn't want another baby so we weren't trying. I made one mistake and was pregnant six months after having the second baby, but I miscarried. About seven months after that, I made another mistake and got pregnant again. So I went from not being able to get pregnant at all, to making two mistakes and getting pregnant both times. There were times when I doubted I'd ever have a family, and I would never have believed I would end up with three children. It was a very happy ending. Having thought I would never have children, I will never take them for granted.

'It changed me, definitely. I don't know if it would have been the case anyway, but my family comes first in my life. I was quite focused on work before, but now I put a huge amount of pressure on myself to be the right parent, trying to make sure that everything is done properly. I do know that I put 100 per cent into it.

'Three children is very hard work, but they are good children. People often say that they are very well behaved. That's no piece of cake, and I am very proud of them. They are now eight, six and four. The challenges have changed, and now it is the juggling of so many things. I do moan sometimes with the daily grind of it all and I do have bad days, but it was all worth it. I've had friends who have never been able to have children and I think that's so awful that I never want to take my own children for granted. Even on bad days I try not to take them for granted, and to put a lot of effort into them. I am a bit of a perfectionist about it. They mean the world to me and I was very lucky.

'I love all my children equally but there is something very special about my first, who was an IVF baby. She is the most level-headed, mature, diligent child and a lot of people say how wonderful she is and that there is something unique about her. She has been like that from the word go, she is such a lovely person. After all the effort we had to get her, it is rewarding. She doesn't know she was an IVF baby. She's eight and a half now, but she's not like my six-year-old who questions everything. She does know that it took a long time for her to come and that she was a very wanted baby. She's not really aware of the facts of life yet, but I know that before she goes to middle school I will tell her, we will have that conversation. I think it is important that she does know, but I don't think it will make any difference.

'I used to advise about nutrition, and I did enjoy my job, but when I had the children it wasn't what I wanted. I used to switch off. I just thought I couldn't be doing it, and then I stopped working. I became a parent-governor on a whim and went into school on some visits and I really enjoyed being around children. It just went from there really and I am doing teaching assistant work. Initially I was thinking of teaching, but it's too much at the moment so I thought I would start from that.

'We were lucky that this really strengthened our relation-ship, although to start with I did feel very alone as my husband was totally switched off. He couldn't cope and wasn't ready for it, or very supportive. He will say now that the most important thing is to communicate. He saw the pressure that going through IUI put me under and that was when it changed for him. We have got a good friend-ship within our relationship. We are both very down to earth and good at communicating. Having small children does put pressure on you though, and it's something you have to work at.'

CHAPTER 8

Trying Again

Having experienced parenthood and all the joys that a child can bring, it is natural that you will start thinking about trying to have another baby at some point. If you know that you are going to need treatment, you may want to get started fairly soon, particularly if you are older or are very aware of your biological clock ticking away; however, you may want to allow yourself some time to get over the rocky road that has led through a prolonged period of infertility, followed by the roller-coaster of treatment and then all the highs and lows of pregnancy, birth and early parenthood.

It is not uncommon for people to feel ambiguous about the whole idea of trying fertility treatment again. Having finally escaped from what has often been a hugely traumatic experience of infertility, the thought of going back to the clinic and starting all over again, with no guarantee of another positive outcome, can be daunting. This time it will not just be you and your partner to consider when thinking about treatment, but also your young child, and you may decide that you would rather enjoy life as you are rather than going through more pain and angst in order to try to enlarge your family.

Secondary infertility (that's infertility when you have conceived in the past) is not as obviously painful as primary infertility (when you're trying for a first child). You are no longer childless and wondering whether you will ever have a family, but you are now a parent. People often assume that it must be much easier for couples who are trying for a second child, but secondary infertility can bring a whole new set of issues and unique difficulties of its own.

How soon can I start trying again?

Pregnancy, birth and breastfeeding all have a huge impact on your hormones, and you can't start IVF again until your body has recovered from this. Most women who have tried for some time to get pregnant are keen to breastfeed if they possibly can, and you will need to wait until you have stopped breastfeeding before you start more treatment. Breastfeeding will have an effect on your periods, and they may take a while to return to normal. Some women find that they start having periods again when they are still breastfeeding, but for others their menstrual cycle won't return until a month or two after they've stopped feeding their baby. If you do have periods while you are breastfeeding, they may be longer or shorter than normal and are sometimes irregular.

For many women who've had fertility treatment, age is often the most important factor when making a decision about how long to leave it before returning to the clinic.

Fertility treatment is less successful for older women, and if you are already in your forties or approaching 40, you will probably want to start treatment sooner rather than later if you'd like to try to have another child. Women sometimes feel pressured into having more treatment far sooner than they would really like to just because they are worried that their chances of success are rapidly diminishing with age. You will need to weigh up the desire for another child against the need to have time to enjoy your first baby without the pressure of more fertility treatment. Younger women may be happy to wait much longer before even thinking about treatment, in order to have some time and space with their existing child.

'I'm just 40 now and I know I am lucky to have a baby at all, but I'd really love to have a bigger family. My son is only seven months old and it has been so great to have him, but I don't feel there is time to enjoy it because there is this pressure to get on with more treatment. Every month I leave it, it's less likely to work. There's no getting away from that, and I am so torn. I'd like to just forget all about it like a normal person would, but I can't.'   *Rebecca*

The expert view
Professor Bill Ledger, University of New South Wales

'I think it is really important that the couple give time to their baby. They've been very fortunate to have a child through IVF and it deserves time. Giving some love

continued

and some time to that young child until he or she is at least a year old seems reasonable to me. I've had people who have deliberately not breastfed because they have wanted to get on and start ovulating again because of this smoking gun of female ageing. We sometimes over-emphasise the impact of age on fertility. It is important, but bonding with your child is also important and there is a balance to be struck.'

Financial considerations

Although there is some funded fertility treatment for couples who are trying to conceive their first child, there is not usually any help for those who want a second or third child. If you got pregnant first time around after taking fertility drugs or having IUI, cost may not be a big issue, but IVF or ICSI are expensive treatments and often involve a hefty bill for drugs too. This can come as a shock to anyone who had funded treatment the first time around. Of course, if you have frozen embryos left over from previous treatment, having them transferred will not be as expensive as starting another fresh cycle.

You should think carefully about how much money you are willing and able to spend when you are making a decision about trying for another child. If you are only going to be able to afford one cycle, you need to be realistic about the chances of success. Getting pregnant once after IVF will certainly give you a better prognosis for further treatment, but it doesn't automatically follow that you will be able to get pregnant again.

Many couples are denied the chance to have a second child because they simply can't afford to pay for more treatment. Others decide that they would rather spend any spare cash they do have on ensuring that all their existing child's needs are met. It is tough if you are denied the opportunity to try to have a second child on financial grounds, but unfortunately this is a reality for many couples.

'Because they said that they couldn't find anything wrong, I was hoping I might fall pregnant naturally after having a baby, but I haven't and we don't know whether we will ever have the money to do IVF again. I did enquire about having funding on the NHS again but a lot of people don't get funded at all and have to pay for it, and I felt I was being a bit greedy. We have spoken about egg sharing, but what puts me off is that a child could find out about it when they were 18. That is a bit of a worry because if we never have another child, I don't think I could cope if we found out there was one somewhere from one of my eggs. We said no to that straight away.'
Kelly

Might it be possible for me to get pregnant again naturally?

We've all heard stories of people who spent years trying to get pregnant and then after eventually conceiving with IVF, went on to have another child, or two, naturally. Younger women and those with minor or unexplained fertility problems are the most likely to conceive naturally after fertility treatment, but sometimes even those with more complex issues can get pregnant without more medical assistance after a first pregnancy. During pregnancy, your body changes hugely both physically and hormonally, and this can kick-start something which makes it possible for pregnancy to occur naturally in the future.

I'd heard so many tales of miraculous second conceptions, that I couldn't help hoping it might happen to me. I would have been a fairly good candidate for a possible natural pregnancy after having a first IVF baby, being (at the time) on the right side of 35 with unexplained infertility. We're so often told that hectic lifestyles, busy careers and stress can cause fertility problems and once I was at home with my baby, eating healthily and enjoying life, and feeling relaxed and happy if a little sleep-deprived, I felt certain that these must be the optimum conditions for a natural conception. We did leave it for a couple of years before resigning ourselves to the fact that we'd have to go through more IVF if we wanted another child, but it does show that getting rid of the stress in your life is not necessarily a solution to unexplained infertility!

There are some people who do get pregnant naturally despite having had tubal or hormonal problems that made it seem virtually impossible. It can happen, and it does happen, but it isn't worth waiting years 'just in case' you have a natural conception if you are getting older and your chances of success with fertility treatment are dwindling.

The expert view

Professor Bill Ledger, University of New South Wales

'It's not uncommon that a woman will have a natural pregnancy after an IVF pregnancy, depending on the cause in the first place. Pregnancy changes a woman's physiology quite dramatically and things don't go back to the way they were. We see people who didn't ovulate naturally who then ovulate after the child is born, people who have got adhesions in the pelvis and tubal damage who sometimes get pregnant naturally after the uterus and tubes are reorganised because of the growing baby.

'Your chance of getting pregnant naturally depends on the severity of your fertility problem. It is more common after unexplained infertility, and younger people with unexplained infertility will sometimes conceive naturally after IVF. If you've got a profound tubal blockage, then that is unlikely to reverse, but someone who has a milder degree of tubal damage can have a natural pregnancy sometimes if the problem wasn't absolute. It's partly due to pregnancy and the pregnancy hormones but also the amazing anatomical changes when your uterus goes from the size of a large plum to the size of a full-term baby – it is the most remarkable change in any structure in the body in the whole of your life and it is not surprising therefore that when the pregnancy is over the anatomy doesn't change back to where it was before.'

Clare's story

Clare and Matt had been trying for a baby for five years before they had their son, Alex, after their third IVF attempt. The first two attempts had ended in miscarriage. Clare had blocked Fallopian tubes, and so the couple were certain they would never be able to conceive naturally. When Alex was seven and a half months old, Clare began to feel unwell.

'I was feeling really sick and tired and I thought I was ill. I'd actually booked an appointment to go and see the doctor because I couldn't understand why I felt the way I did – I just felt dreadful and constantly nauseous, but it never occurred to me that I could be pregnant. We thought it was utterly impossible that we would have another child naturally, as both my tubes were completely blocked.

'The day before my doctor's appointment, I was in the kitchen having a cup of tea and looking at my calendar and I suddenly started putting dates together. I thought, *Hang on a minute – I feel sick in the mornings when I wake up, I'm really tired, maybe I'm not ill*. My husband came home 20 minutes later and I said that I thought I might be pregnant. He just looked at me with a 'you've completely lost your marbles' kind of look and said I could discuss it at the doctor's appointment the next morning. I said he had to be joking, as there was no way I was going to go to sleep that night if I didn't find out once the idea had been planted in my head. I ended up dashing out that night to the supermarket to get a pregnancy test. It came up pregnant straight away.

'I was absolutely euphoric, but obviously very nervous at the same time, because I'd had two miscarriages prior to

Alex and we'd also been warned that if I got pregnant there was a high risk of it being ectopic because of the state of my tubes.

'My doctor was stunned and he referred me to the consultant at the hospital just to check that it wasn't ectopic – in fact, the appointment didn't come through until I was 20 weeks pregnant, which would have been a bit late if it had been an ectopic. A few weeks after I found out that I was pregnant, I had bad pains in my shoulder and travelling up my right side and I really did think that I had an ectopic. So we went to our local hospital and had a scan. They did find that the pregnancy was definitely uterine, but it was too early to say whether it was a viable pregnancy. They asked us to go back two weeks later and I had a horrendous scan where they measured the wrong heartbeat – the doctor thought my heartbeat was the baby's heartbeat and told us that the pregnancy would end in miscarriage.

'I phoned my IVF consultant absolutely distraught. She is amazing and she said that they would do a scan and would look after us. We had the scan and she found the heartbeat right away and said it was a viable pregnancy and she was just absolutely stunned. I asked her how on earth it had happened, and she said she didn't understand. She said she had seen the state of my tubes and she couldn't explain how the baby had arrived there.

'I have no idea what the percentages are for the number of women who have a baby through IVF and then conceive naturally, but I have since discovered that there are a fair number. I'd be interested to know, because for everyone like me, there's another dozen who have never been able to have another child or have had to have more treatment.'

Going back to the clinic

Once you have decided that you want to try more fertility treatment, you need to think about where you will go for this. There are many advantages to going back to the same clinic, as the staff there will have all your notes and will be familiar with the way that you have responded during previous treatment. Sometimes this isn't practical, particularly if you have moved home or if the funding situation dictated where you had to go first time around. Some couples who didn't have a particularly good experience during earlier treatment cycles may prefer not to go back to the same clinic.

If you are choosing a new clinic, do your research thoroughly before making a decision, looking not just at success rates but also the cost of treatment and what is offered, as well as the location. This can be particularly important once you have a child, as you will need to think about how you will manage this with visits to the clinic.

Book an appointment to go and talk to one of the doctors at the clinic before you start again. They will be able to look through your notes (make sure you get your notes to take with you to a new clinic if you are moving from one to another) to see how things went in your previous treatment and to discuss how your treatment will be managed.

Finding yourself back at the fertility clinic can bring a range of emotions which may take you by surprise. For the past year or so, you have been submerged in the world of babies and parenting, and being back at the clinic can sometimes feel as if you are taking a step backwards and may dredge up feelings you haven't experienced for some time, so do be prepared for this.

Is it all right to take my child to the fertility clinic with me?

It is not always possible to arrange childcare if you have numerous visits to the fertility clinic, and clinic staff accept that people may sometimes need to bring their children with them. There are two ways of thinking about this. Some people believe that having children in the waiting room gives hope and optimism to those who haven't yet been successful, others feel that it is painful and upsetting. If you have to take your child with you to the clinic, try to be as sensitive to how other people might feel about this as you can.

Should we tell our child that we are trying to have another baby?

What you tell your child about your treatment will depend in part on how old she is when you start trying. With a younger child, you may not need to say anything at all, but an older child may have started to ask questions about the possibility of having a sibling, and it may be more difficult to conceal frequent visits to the clinic and discussions about treatment with your partner.

If you are going to tell your child, there are a number

of factors to bear in mind. Don't do it unless you are quite happy for all and sundry to find out about it – young children tend to find it impossible to keep secrets, and you may discover that your child's friends and teachers, as well as the next-door neighbours and the milkman, all know that you are trying for another baby. Do make sure that you explain to your child that having a brother or sister is not an inevitability. If you have told her how she was conceived, she may assume that fertility treatment always works, and if you haven't, she has no reason to think that you won't be able to have another baby. Dealing with your child's disappointment as well as your own can be really tough, so try to make it clear that having a brother or sister would be nice, but that you're very happy to have her as your only child.

My son was three when we were having treatment and had started to ask questions about the possibility of siblings. I explained that it wasn't easy for us to have babies and that we had to get a doctor to help us. I told him we'd been very lucky to have him, and that although we would try to make him a baby brother or sister, it might not be possible. He went off to play looking thoughtful. It was a month or two before Christmas, and we'd been talking about all the Christmas presents and decorations which had started appearing in the shops, so I probably shouldn't have been surprised when he came back a little later having solved our fertility problem. 'It's all right Mummy,' he said, patting me gently on the back. 'Don't worry about getting a baby. I'm sure there will be lots of babies in the shops for Christmas.'

Do most people get pregnant again if they've already had a baby?

Your chances of having a baby after fertility treatment are certainly higher if you've already conceived a first child that way, and many couples do go on to have a second, or even a third child after treatment; however, your circumstances and your age also help determine the chances of a positive outcome. If you are younger and have good-quality eggs and your partner has good-quality sperm, you are more likely to get pregnant. If you had your first baby when you were in your forties and have a low ovarian reserve with some male factor issues too, your chances of success will not be so good.

One possibly cheering fact is that statistics show that your chances of getting pregnant with fertility treatment are higher if you've had treatment first time around than if you got pregnant naturally with your previous child. I was initially quite surprised by that, until it was explained that if you've had a baby after fertility treatment, then you know the treatment can work for you, as it has managed to successfully override your fertility problem in the past. So, for once, infertility actually puts you ahead of the game. Of course, having had a child doesn't guarantee that treatment will work again for you, but it certainly boosts your chances of success.

How many treatment cycles should you try before giving up?

There is often a natural limit to the number of cycles a couple can tolerate emotionally and financially before they consider giving up on treatment, but the point at which this limit is reached will not be the same for everyone. If you can afford more treatment and the medical team treating you think that there is a reasonable chance of success, you may want to carry on for as many cycles as you can comfortably fund. If you are being told that the chances of a positive outcome are very low, you may want to stop sooner rather than later.

The expert view

Professor Bill Ledger, University of New South Wales

'We like to look at each case individually. If you have someone who has had an IVF baby and their second cycle goes well but they don't have a pregnancy despite having good embryos, then it is worthwhile carrying on. On the other hand, when the woman has become older while raising the first baby, and then she has a cycle with only one or two eggs which don't fertilise, then I think there is a message there. That's when people should stop, because their body is not responding the way it should do and giving them a high chance of pregnancy.'

Trying more invasive treatment

Sometimes, women who have got pregnant the first time around with a low-tech fertility treatment, such as a course of drugs, may find that they need more invasive treatment in order to conceive again. In most situations, it makes sense to begin by trying what has been successful for you in the past, but problems arise if the treatment doesn't seem to be having the same effect second time around. Age can be particularly relevant here, as a solution to a minor fertility problem when you were in your mid-thirties may not work for the same problem if you are older.

It can be hard to decide how long you should carry on with the same treatment before moving up a notch to something that may be more effective but is also likely to be more expensive, invasive and stressful. You should discuss your options carefully with your consultant and weigh up the pros and cons before making a decision.

Using frozen embryos

If you have frozen embryos from a previous treatment cycle, then having a frozen embryo transfer will be considerably cheaper than having to start a fresh cycle. It is also less invasive, as you don't have to have egg collection and you won't require as many drugs as you did for a fresh cycle, if you need any at all. Don't forget that not all embryos will survive the freezing and thawing process, and that you may not end up with as many to transfer as you have expected.

It is increasingly common to keep embryos in culture for longer, because if they can survive for five days to reach blastocyst stage, the chances of successful implantation are higher. This means that fewer embryos are frozen, as not all embryos will survive this long in the laboratory. The pregnancy rate from frozen blastocysts is higher than that from an embryo that has been frozen on day two or three.

You may not be sure that you will be able to use all your frozen embryos if you have a fair number of them. Couples who have had twins, or who have had a difficult time during pregnancy and birth, may be ambivalent as to whether they really want another child. Making the decision not to continue to keep your embryos in storage can be very tough, and some couples choose to leave them for as long as they can to avoid making the decision. Your embryos can only be stored for a set period, however, and your clinic will get in touch with you to let you know when they are close to the end of that time. You will then have to make a final decision as to whether you are going to use them or not. You may need some expert advice or counselling at this point if you are uncertain and feeling torn. If you don't want to use the embryos yourself, you may choose to donate them to another couple, to allow them to be used for research projects or to let them perish.

Is it easier to cope with fertility treatment second time around?

The raw pain of childlessness no longer overwhelms you when you are having treatment in order to have another child. You know that you are fortunate, you know that you should be grateful that you've been successful, but you also know that going through fertility treatment is never an easy business.

Although you are no longer worrying about facing a childless future and the possibility of never having a family, there are some additional concerns when you are in this position. You know what an amazing experience it is to have a child of your own and you know what you are missing out on by not being able to do it again. You may desperately want your son or daughter to have a sibling and feel that you are somehow failing them by not being able to make another baby.

When you already have a child, you can't escape babies and pregnant women in the way that you could when you were childless. Your child's friends' parents may all be talking about having another baby; they may already be expecting or may have younger children. Every time you take your child to a playgroup, to nursery or to school, you will be faced with bumps and babies. It can be more difficult to be rational about this when you can't avoid pregnant women and young children.

The other difficulty with secondary infertility is often the lack of support and understanding. When you are trying for a first child, friends and family will generally be sympathetic. Once you have a child, people may be far less supportive if you find it difficult to cope. Some may suggest that you ought to be grateful for what you have, rather than fussing about what you don't have. If you had found solace in a fertility support group first time around, it may seem inappropriate to go along to a meeting now to talk about how you are feeling when the other people there are childless. Some people say that they feel greedy for wanting another child when they're in the fertility clinic waiting room, surrounded by childless couples. Try to remember that wanting another child is a perfectly legitimate desire. There are online forums and support networks for those experiencing secondary infertility and it is a good idea to seek these out – you will find details at the end of this book.

The expert view
Professor Bill Ledger, University of New South Wales

'In one way it is easier doing it again, because you know what the process involves, so you are not taking the step into the unknown that people who are doing the first cycle or who haven't had a pregnancy are – so you are in a better position to make an informed decision about whether you want to do it again. You need to decide whether you really want to put yourself through it all again – it is stressful and difficult, you do have a child, you can have a happy family life. Don't be driven by what other people want, make sure it is your own decision that you have made as a couple and that it is what you really want to do.

'The other thing I would stress if you are going to have a second IVF attempt is that you should have a single embryo transfer. I think someone who has had a baby through IVF should consider single embryo transfer

continued

and freezing any other embryos. If you bring twins into the world with an older sibling, that older sibling's life is going to be affected because you will spend so much of your life looking after the twins.'

When treatment doesn't work

Sometimes you will reach a point where you have to accept that treatment isn't going to work. It can be particularly frustrating when you've had successful treatment in the past, as you will have gone into it full of hope and expectation. The point at which you decide to stop is an individual decision, and it might be influenced by your finances, your age or the stress you have experienced during treatment.

You should recognise the pain and upset you feel at not being able to have another child. It is easy to say that you should be grateful because you already have one child, but if you have always wanted a larger family, it is difficult to let go of that dream. Feeling sad about this is valid, and you need to accept this in order to be able to move on.

Adoption and fostering

You may wish to consider adoption as an alternative way forward if you can't have another child through treatment. You can adopt if you have an existing child, but this is not something to be undertaken without a great deal of thought and preparation. The most important person to consider when you are thinking about this is your existing child. Your family dynamic would change quite suddenly, and having been the focus of your attention, your child could feel usurped. Many of the children who need adoptive families have been through very tough times, and they can be quite challenging. You would need to think about the impact this would have on your child.

Adoption takes time, as an adoption agency would want to be absolutely certain that you are the right family for a child, so this is not going to be an instant solution to your desire to expand your family. Your child will also have to have reached a certain age before an adoption agency would consider you as prospective adoptive parents, as they like to keep an age gap between children in a family.

Fostering is another alternative, but this is generally a short-term measure, offering a temporary home to a child. Again, you would need to think very carefully about the effect this would have on your child, as it will not necessarily be easy. You would not be able to foster a child close in age to your own child.

If you are interested in fostering or adoption, it is essential that you spend some time looking into what would be involved first. You can find useful contacts at the back of the book.

Anya's story

Anya and Damion's first child, a daughter Hope, was born against the odds after ICSI as they'd been told it was unlikely they would ever have a child of their own.

'We'd always talked about having three or four kids, and right from the outset, even before we were married, we'd talked about big families. Hope was just past her first birthday when we started trying again. Our odds to get her had been so ridiculously bad that I went into it quite cautiously. The first cycle after Hope, we did have a biochemical pregnancy but it was a really low reading, and a couple of days later I started bleeding. We had three failed cycles before Barney.

'The hard bit was juggling with Hope. I didn't work at the time, so she just came along with me and I did my best to make it a nice outing. We said right from the start that Hope wasn't going to suffer because we were going to try for number two. She came with me to the clinic and crawled around and she was part of it. I don't think I spent any less time with her than I would have done.

'I think secondary infertility is very isolating, very misunderstood and really, really painful. You go from the abstract longing for the child, from thinking it would be amazing, to knowing that actually it really is amazing – there's nothing that tops being a parent. You have this picture in your head of what a family looks like and you are not quite there. I was totally bowled over that I had Hope, and it was a miracle, but that didn't stop me desperately wanting a sibling for her, and the two emotions can go hand in hand. It was a terrible struggle to go through and she was a comfort, obviously, but the sadness was still very real. You are surrounded by people who have got number two very easily. People can be there when you are trying for the first one, but they have their own lives and they get tired. We had Barney on cycle number five, and it was meant to be our last one. It did take its toll. We had talked about it and we were going to look at adoption if it didn't work.

'I really would love a third child. When we were going through secondary infertility, it felt as if there was a hole in our lives. Now it feels as if we have room in our lives and there's potential. We've got emotional reserves and the kids would love a sibling, so all of those things make me feel that it would be lovely, but if it doesn't happen I don't feel unfulfilled like I did with secondary infertility. I know that I would be able to let go now that we are a family of four, whereas when we were a family of three, I didn't feel like a family, I felt like a parent.

'We are looking at adoption now or even doing IVF over the next year or so. Worries about how adoption would affect Hope and Barney is a reason that we'd look at IVF rather than adoption. My biggest fear is not that my husband and I couldn't handle adoption, it's that the child could have big issues and be jealous of my kids or something. I'd hate the children to be adversely affected. If it looks like that might be too big an issue then we either say that we've now got our family, or we'd do IVF again. If we did it again, we'd probably do two cycles, and then draw a line under it.

'I can completely understand the arguments for just stopping, but I think that while there is a question we do have to think about it. I wouldn't expect much support from people, because they are right in some ways that we have spent an awful lot of time, money and effort to get the two children so why not just stop? But while there is still a chance, we are not quite ready to give up.'

CHAPTER 9

An Only Child

When it has taken some time to get pregnant, your situation may end up limiting the size of your family. Whether it's because you know that you are not likely to be able to get pregnant again, because you can't face having more fertility treatment, are too old to try again or simply don't have the money, your family size may be dictated by this and you may not be able to have more than one child. For some people, achieving the long-awaited goal of having a child is quite enough and they are perfectly happy to have just one, but for others this may involve some readjustment of the hopes and dreams about their future family.

There are all kinds of negative stereotypes about only children and parents who only have one child. As parents, you may feel that people assume you aren't willing to change your life enough to have more children, that you are somehow selfish or too concerned about your finances. Only children are often assumed to be spoilt, selfish and precocious, and may be considered bossy, aggressive and antisocial. It can be very distressing if you feel that other people are judging your family because you have one child and making assumptions that are simply incorrect. Of course, some only children may be spoilt and bossy, but so are some children with siblings. Most research suggests that there are not such big differences between only children and those from larger families, and there may be some positive side effects from being an only child, as this will certainly have benefits for your child financially and materially.

Being an only child is becoming a more common experience for children growing up in many countries around the world. In the UK around a quarter of children are growing up without siblings, and in some other parts of Europe the percentages are higher, while in China, where there has been a one-child-only policy, the majority of the younger generation are growing up as only children.

The expert view

Dr Bernice Sorensen, psychotherapist specialising in only children

'I don't think there is any fundamental difference between only children and those with siblings, but I do think being brought up as an only child is a different experience. And because it is a different experience, you begin to see the world in a different way. It's not right or wrong – just different. There are positives to being an only child, but they are primarily economic and we live in a society where actually that is a really big plus. I don't think people should have an extra child just because they think that they have got to provide a sibling – I don't think that is necessary.'

Dealing with your own disappointment

When you'd envisaged your future, you may have always imagined a family with at least two children. Once you've had a child, you may be left longing for another, to provide your child with a sibling and adjust the balance of your family. You may be very aware that you should feel grateful that you have managed to have a child at all, you know how much other couples still trying unsuccessfully to conceive would long to be in your shoes, but that doesn't stop you wanting a bigger family. Now you have seen what joy a child can bring to your life, you know what you are missing out on by not being able to do it again.

There are many reasons why people may not be able to have another child, and that can make a difference to how you manage. If you have been told that it would be impossible for you to get pregnant again or you know that your body would not be able to deal with another pregnancy, this may be very difficult to cope with initially but with time you will probably reach a point of acceptance. If you know you simply couldn't handle more treatment and have decided that it would be unfair to put your existing family through this, then you have made an active decision about this which you will be able to come to terms with. It is sometimes far more difficult to feel contented if it is only finances that stand between you and more treatment, or if you feel it is your own fault for having left it too late to try for a child which has left you in a position where you will never be able to do this again.

'I don't like people getting the idea that it's a lifestyle choice only having one child. I'd love him to have a brother or sister. I always thought I'd have four children; I never really wanted only one. I am happy with one child but I think I'd feel complete with two. I would go through treatment again – definitely – but at the moment there is no chance financially.'

Alice

Dealing with other people

People do sometimes make assumptions about single-child families and may conclude that you must have decided that work or money were more important to you than having more children, or even that you are in some way selfish. They often have no qualms about asking why you didn't want to have more children, and the way you deal with this will depend on how open you are about your fertility problems. It can feel as if even your experiences of family life are somehow still coloured by your past, and that makes it harder to put this behind you. You will find as your child gets older that you are no longer plagued by the 'when are you going to have another one?' questions and that will start to make it easier.

My child wants a sibling

Many people who have an only child say that one of the issues that causes them most sadness is not being able to provide their child with a sibling. If your child is old enough to start asking questions, they will inevitably at some point want to know why they don't have a brother or sister. If you are feeling upset about this yourself, your child's questions may take on an added significance and you may assume that your child is as distressed about not having a sibling as you are about not having another child. If you think about it, your child may have actually asked more often why you can't have a dog or a rabbit, or why you can't spend every holiday at Disneyland, but you are unlikely to feel that these things are a source of deprivation yourself and so may not take them as seriously.

Children don't like being different, and if your child is surrounded by friends who have siblings, this can make him feel that he isn't the same as everyone else. If you can ensure that he mixes with some other only children too, he will soon realise that being an only child is not particularly unusual, and that he doesn't need to feel that he is in any way abnormal.

It's important to be realistic about the fact that although children may talk about how much they'd like a sibling, the reality of having a brother or sister is not always the wonderful experience they are imagining. Your child would like a younger brother or sister who will play games, share their interests and be happy to tag along playing second fiddle, but a new baby is often a great disappointment to older siblings. Babies are noisy and demanding, they take up lots of parental time and attention and they are rather dull if what you'd been hoping for was a playmate. Even as they grow older, although there will be many joys, there will also be much squabbling, sibling rivalry and endless arguments.

You may feel guilty about having deprived your child of the fun of having a sibling, but remember that he is used to being an only and this is his normality. If you are forever worried that he is somehow at a disadvantage, you will convey some of this anxiety to your child. If you can accept the situation and focus on the positives, the chances are that your child will be able to do this too.

Allowing your child to have independence

When you have only one child you may feel that you worry more than other parents, and you may suspect that you can be rather overprotective at times. It may be hard to leave your child with other people or to let him have as much independence as his peers. It is sometimes hard to overcome feelings of fear that something awful could happen to your child, but try to remember that this is just part of being a parent. Your child needs to feel that you trust him and that you can allow him the independence to grow and to develop as an individual.

You may also find it more difficult to keep any problems your child encounters in perspective. Children often come home from school relating tales of great injustice and unfairness from their peers, and it is easy to become very upset or concerned at what your child is telling you. Left to his own devices, he may have entirely forgotten about it by the next day, but if you get involved and try to sort things out on his behalf, this can exacerbate the problem. Girls' friendships can be particularly poisonous when they are young, and they are forever switching allegiances or leaving one another out. It may all sound quite dreadful to you as an adult, but it is best not to jump in too quickly to try to smooth the waters. Sometimes adults reflect their own insecurities onto their children, and if you don't always feel socially confident that may make you more concerned about any problems your child seems to be having. Remember that children have to learn to fight their own battles, and these playground disputes are all part of learning how to be a sociable adult.

Demolishing the myths

Many of the stereotypes that have built up around only children are in part what parents find so difficult to deal with. Parents of only children worry that their child will be spoilt or lonely, that they may grow up finding it difficult to relate to others or to have a relationship. If you think about the adults you know who were only children, you will probably realise fairly quickly that this is not the case and that many perfectly normal, stable, balanced adults don't have any siblings. The stereotypes may have some grounding in reality, but positive parenting has far more of an influence on your child's development.

Only children are spoilt Of course, only children will get more parental attention, but that doesn't mean they are inevitably spoilt by this. It all depends on the type of attention you give them, and how you deal with them. If you give your child everything he wants the moment he wants it, then he may very well end up spoilt – but this rule applies to children who have siblings in just the same way. It's the parental attitude, not the fact of being an only, that makes the difference.

Only children are selfish The idea that children who have siblings all share things happily is not true, as often sibling rivalry can make it harder for children who come from large families to feel happy about sharing things. Very young children find it difficult to share, but if you teach your child how to share with others and show him that this will mean others will share with him, there is no reason at all for an only child to be any more selfish than anyone else.

Only children are lonely Most only children are quite good at being by themselves because they will have more time alone than those with siblings; however, being alone and being lonely are two very different concepts, and as long as you ensure that your child spends time with other children, this does not need to be a problem. In fact, the ability to be content in your own company is often a very useful life skill.

Only children can't make friends Sometimes, if only children spend all their time in the company of adults, they can find it difficult to relate to other children of their own age, but this is an exception, not a rule. It is down to you as a parent to make sure your child spends time with others of his own age, and to give him some space and freedom to do this.

'Our son is going to be an only child and I need to find the positives. I don't want him to be mollycoddled and spoilt. Someone said to me that because he was my only child and he was IVF, he was obviously spoilt and I was really offended by that. I want him to be brought up properly with good values and I am paranoid about spoiling him. In some ways I am quite hard on him, maybe I'm harder because I am over-compensating for the fact that I might spoil him.'   *Sophie*

How to avoid problems

Most parents of only children are only too aware of the potential problems that their children can face if they over-indulge them, and do make an effort to set boundaries and to be firm when this is necessary. It seems that one of the most important things is to ensure that an only child gets used to the rough and tumble of being with their peers by spending plenty of time with other children. The stereo-typical image of the spoilt, precocious only child can often be put down to spending too much time with adults and not enough with other children, which is easily avoided.

The expert view

Dr Bernice Sorensen, psychotherapist specialising in only children

'One of the difficulties is when children mostly have adult input. They are used to having a very special place which

continued

---

they are not going to have with their peers, or even with other adults, because other adults aren't half as indulgent as parents normally are. If children mostly have adult attention they do get a sense of themselves as much more important than they are – a sort of gran-diosity. When they go to school, they act like little adults and that's why a lot of only children get bullied. It's common because they haven't had the advantage of having social skills that siblings enable you to learn. But it's not inevitable because you can make sure that your child has other children to play with. To me that is so pivotal but most people don't really take that terribly seriously.'

Dr Sorensen has put together a checklist for parents of only children, to ensure that being an only is a positive experience for your child and to avoid some of the pitfalls that parents of only children can sometimes fall into.

- Don't overcompensate with too many 'goodies'. Only children have to put up with enough envy without making it worse.
- Don't tell them that they are lucky not to have siblings, even if you believe it. It may be true for you but don't assume your child has the same feelings.
- Make sure your child has plenty of children to play with and to stay with.
- Let them be a child, not a little adult.

- Make a big effort to let them separate from you psychologically, and this may also mean financially, as they get into their teens.
- Encourage them to join groups and clubs.
- Make sure they go to mixed-sex schools.
- Don't overprotect them or expect too much independence too early.
- Don't expect them to fulfil your thwarted ambitions.
- Ensure you do not become enmeshed with them.
- Remember your child will be much more sensitive to your needs than children who have siblings are to their parents, so let them know you have a life outside of them.
- Make them wait for things or you will set up expectations of instant gratification, which is hard for them to unlearn once they have relationships.
- Teach them how to share – not with you but with other children.

A positive experience

Being an only child can be a very positive experience, as there are financial and material advantages that can make life easier and more fulfilling. Indeed, some recent research suggested that only children are actually happier and that the more siblings a child has, the less happy they are. The key message to successfully raising an only child seems to be not to focus too much on your child and to try not to expect too much of them, but rather to let them grow in their own way and to enjoy seeing the paths that they choose in life.

You may have preferred to have a larger family, but many couples nowadays actively choose to have just one child and this is becoming ever more common. Families where there is just one child tend to have a very close bond between them, and adults who have grown up as only children are often positive about their experiences. They know that they have had opportunities that would not otherwise have been possible, and only children are often self-confident, independent high-achievers who do very well in life.

Diana's story

Diana and Mark had their daughter after ICSI treatment, and she is their only child.

'If we hadn't been through this, things would be different. We would have had our daughter earlier so we would have been a lot younger, and there would probably have been more than one. We did try again, but it didn't work. They defrosted the embryos and they were all damaged – there was nothing that they could put back, so we never got as far as transfer. If I am absolutely honest, at that time, although I was upset, I felt that if we hadn't had the embryos, we wouldn't have done it again. I don't think we would have started from scratch again. At that point we thought *Be thankful for what you have got*. It was a fairly easy decision. In some ways, with hindsight I enjoyed her so much when she was younger that I could not ever

imagine having another child that I would love so much.
For her, I think it would have been nice to have a brother
or sister

'My philosophy on it now is that life is not perfect – you
don't know what is round the corner so I try not to dwell
on it. If we had two, we couldn't send her to the school
that she goes to, she wouldn't have the life that she leads
and we wouldn't be the parents that we are. You make
the best of what there is.

'Quite a lot of our friends have got one child, either
because they have chosen that or because of their situations, so in the group we are in, there are quite a few
people with just one child. My daughter is starting to ask
about it now because everybody in her class has a brother
or sister, but some of them have brothers and sisters who
are in their twenties – they might have stepsisters, or their
parents have split up. I don't think that there is any family
formula now in the way that there used to be when I
grew up.

'When she was very small we made her very aware of
the fact that she was an IVF baby. She knows that we tried
really hard and that somebody helped us to have a baby.
Next year she starts doing reproduction at school so I
think we will get more questions. Even within her class,
there are quite a few IVF children. I don't really think it's
any huge issue. It's just another bit of information. I think
it is better to make them aware of it rather than it being
a shock to them. It's also the answer to why we don't have
more. She says, "Why won't you have another baby
mummy?", and I say "Well, mummy can't have another baby,"
and that's the end of the conversation. She understands,

and if she starts getting difficult about it, I say "Well, it upsets mummy too," and then she backs off. Last year we went through "Oh please, please can we try again – or can we have a puppy then?" In the end we got a hamster.

'I said to her that you don't always get what you want. She does understand that and she understands that it's not something that happens that easily. One of my friends had a second child when her first one was eight, so there was an eight-year gap between them and after that she started saying, "Could you not just try again?" She said, "You and daddy, can you go and do some cuddling," but I said the cuddling didn't really work either.

'We don't spoil her and I am very firm, but we try and enjoy it as opposed to everything being a task. I'm a very different person now. I do think it changes you – it does give you a very different perspective on life.'

CHAPTER 10

More Than One

Discovering that you are finally pregnant after some years is always quite a shock, but finding out that you are expecting more than one baby can be completely over-whelming. Naturally, just one in every 80 births would be a multiple, but after fertility treatment that rises hugely to one in every four births. In recent years, there have been moves to try to reduce the number of multiple births after treatment and there are far fewer triplet pregnancies, but the twin rate is still fairly high.

If you have a blood test to check whether or not you are pregnant, this can give an early indication that you may be expecting more than one baby, but this can be confirmed at your first scan. Many people say they feel a huge mix of emotions when they get the news. Although you may be overjoyed and very excited, this is often tempered by a great deal of anxiety and concern about the future.

When you are still trying to get pregnant the idea of the instant family can seem very attractive, as there would be no need to ever go through the emotional and financial stress of treatment again. Once you are faced with the reality of a multiple pregnancy, however, you can be suddenly overwhelmed by the potential risks. Carrying more than one baby at the same time is more difficult and your pregnancy will be considered higher risk because of this, but you can be assured that this means you will be monitored more closely throughout your pregnancy. You will have additional appointments and scans, and you are likely to see a consultant more often too.

Different types of multiple pregnancy

Many multiple pregnancies after fertility treatment are the result of more than one egg being produced and fertilised, and more than one embryo being transferred back into the womb. The babies produced from separate embryos will not be identical, and each embryo will be growing in its own individual sac and will have its own placenta. Twins conceived this way are sometimes referred to as fraternal or dizygotic twins.

Identical twins (known as monozygotic twins) are produced when an embryo divides in two after the egg has been fertilised, and it seems that this happens more frequently after fertility treatment than it would naturally. Sometimes identical twins, or triplets, can share a placenta rather than having one each. When this happens there is a risk of twin-to-twin transfusion syndrome, a condition where one of the babies doesn't grow properly because there is an imbalance in the blood flow between them and one twin receives more blood than the other.

If your babies are sharing a placenta, you will be monitored closely during your pregnancy to ensure that this doesn't cause a problem.

Triplet pregnancies are normally the result of three embryos being transferred during treatment, or of two embryos being transferred and one of them dividing so that there are a pair of identical twins and a third baby. Identical triplets are very rare.

During pregnancy

Women who are carrying more than one baby sometimes have more of the early symptoms of pregnancy, as they have higher levels of pregnancy hormones, so you may feel extremely exhausted or nauseous. There can be a greater risk of some common pregnancy complications such as anaemia, hypertension or pre-eclampsia, and this is why your blood pressure and urine will be checked at your appointments to make sure that no problems are arising.

During pregnancy, you should follow the normal lifestyle advice for pregnant women, making sure that you eat properly, get plenty of fluids, avoid alcohol and don't smoke. The greatest danger with a multiple pregnancy is premature labour, but there isn't anything you can do during pregnancy to eliminate this risk other than looking after yourself. It is important to listen to your body. Carrying more than one baby can be exhausting, and if you feel you are getting really tired it is better to slow down and not to push yourself too hard. Perhaps you may find that you need to stop work a little earlier than you might have planned, or that you need some help around the house towards the end of your pregnancy. If you are finding it tough, don't be afraid to ask for support.

Preparing for your babies

With any long-awaited pregnancy, women often feel that they don't want to tempt fate by getting everything ready too far in advance in case something goes wrong. This may be an understandable reaction, but with multiples it is important to start planning earlier, as you may feel too tired and large to spend hours trawling the shops in the latter stages of pregnancy. Sometimes when multiple babies are born early, parents find themselves completely at sea if they haven't got anything ready – starting off on the wrong foot in that way can make it harder to get back on track.

Make sure that you have the basics that you'll need ready, just in case, and if you feel uncomfortable about shopping early, you can always have an online order ready to be delivered when you need it. It's not just things for the babies that you need to get ready, but also for yourself and your home. Try to get the house ready and stock up the cupboards and freezer. In the first few weeks, you will be totally focused on your babies and if you're well stocked and prepared it can make a huge difference, as it's something you won't have to think about. Your midwife may be able to help advise on everything you will need when your babies arrive, and will also be able to let you know about antenatal classes. If you are planning on going to classes, is makes sense to start them earlier than most other pregnant women would to ensure that you don't miss out.

Buying two – or three – of everything can be extremely expensive, so talk to other mothers of multiples about what they found useful and what you might be able to do without. There are many support groups for parents of multiples, and they often have sales of second-hand baby equipment so you may be able to get some hand-me-downs to help keep costs down.

The birth

Multiple births are often premature, with more than half of all twins being delivered before 37 weeks, and the babies are also more likely to be delivered by Caesarean section. Many women assume that they won't be able to have a vaginal delivery if they're expecting more than one baby, but even given the increased Caesarean rate, about half of all twin pregnancies are delivered vaginally. Another common assumption is that the birth will have to be longer or more difficult, but in fact giving birth to more than one baby can actually be easier because the babies tend to be smaller.

If you're expecting more than one baby, you'll have extra scans during the last trimester of pregnancy to check that the babies are still growing properly. During the scans, the medical team caring for you will also be looking carefully at the position of the babies as this will influence the sort of birth that you are likely to have. If the babies are lying sideways, a Caesarean will be more likely, but if the first baby is lying head downwards, then you may be able to have a normal delivery.

Pregnant women often have a clear idea of the sort of birth they'd like, but we know that birth doesn't often stick to plan and that expectations are not always met. It is even more important to be aware of this if you are having more than one baby, and not to be disappointed if the birth isn't exactly as you might have liked it to be. When you've had a really hard time getting pregnant, you may feel that the birth has been affected by your fertility problems too, but you need to be prepared for this with multiples.

The expert view

Professor James Walker, Royal College of Obstetricians and Gynaecologists

'I certainly wouldn't say that all IVF twin pregnancies should be Caesarean sections. It differs from hospital to hospital, but in our unit, particularly if the first baby is presenting with the head, then we would expect these women to deliver normally. You do need to have expertise, because it is the second one you are worried about – which way round it is going to be, whether it needs help to be delivered, etc. If the second one lines up nicely, then it is quite likely that a woman can have a vaginal delivery, delivered by a midwife in a low-risk environment. As long as you've got cavalry outside to come in and deal with any problems that occur, that's fine.'

Premature babies

Twins and triplets are often born early and so it is more common for babies to need to spend some time in a special care baby unit and some will need neonatal intensive care. It can be really difficult when you have spent so long trying to have a child to find that your babies are whisked away as soon as they arrive. It is only normal to feel anxious and concerned, as this isn't the way that most of us imagine we will bond with our babies after birth. How much help your babies will need and how long they spend in hospital will depend on how early they were born and how much they weighed at birth, as smaller, younger babies tend to need the most help.

One recent study found that in nearly half of all twin pregnancies, one of the babies spent time in neonatal intensive care after they were born, so this is a common problem after fertility treatment. The majority of triplets will need special care. It is very upsetting if your babies seem terribly tiny and fragile, and you may not feel able to celebrate their birth if you are constantly anxious about their health. It is also difficult if your babies are in incubators and you aren't able to be physically close to them and to bond in the way you would have liked in the early days. Try to remember that your babies are getting the best possible care and attention when they are in a special unit. For more information about premature babies, see Chapter 4, Birth.

Breastfeeding

In Chapter 5, page 116, I looked at the advantages of breastfeeding, which we know provides the best nutritional start in life for babies, but for some women the prospect of breastfeeding more than one baby can seem very daunting. It is perfectly possible to produce sufficient milk for more than one baby, but you may need some help establishing feeding. Discuss this with your midwife or health visitor, see a breastfeeding counsellor, if necessary, and do take up any offers of support with this.

If your babies are premature, they may need to be fed through a tube at first, but this doesn't mean that you can't express your milk for them. In fact, breast milk can be particularly beneficial for premature babies, and mothers whose babies are in a special-care baby unit or neonatal intensive care often get extra help trying to establish their milk supply so that their babies can have all the advantages breast milk can bring.

Remember that in order to make a success of breastfeeding, you need to be looking after yourself properly so that you can produce good supplies of milk. You should to make sure that you are eating properly, drinking plenty of water and getting some rest. Establishing a routine will probably help when you are trying to feed more than one baby.

If you really do find it all too much and are having difficulty getting feeding established, if you've already had lots of help and advice but still don't feel you are making any headway, don't feel that you are failing if, in the end, you resort to using formula. Most women can breastfeed successfully if they have good support, but everything is more difficult when you have two or three babies, and it is not worth getting really stressed if you just can't do it.

The expert view

Jane Denton, director, The Multiple Births Foundation

'Breast milk is nutritionally the best milk and it also has the advantage that it's cheaper and can often be quicker if the mother does get into a good pattern and is feeding successfully. The key is getting good help and support in those early days when the babies are first born, when they get used to feeding and you get used to how they like to feed, and then develop your feeding patterns from that. Mothers of twins almost always say to us that the way they cope is to have a routine with them. The mother may choose to feed both babies together but you don't have to do that, there are no hard-and-fast rules at all about it – it is really doing what suits you and the babies the best.'

Building up a support network

Parents, and especially mothers, who've had twins or triplets often say that one of the most useful things they did when they were preparing for their babies was to join a twins or triplets club. Meeting other mothers of multiples is by far the best way of getting an accurate insight into what to expect, and of establishing a support network for the future. The huge increase in the number of multiple births in recent years due to the expansion of fertility treatment means that there are some excellent sources of information and support available, and it is far easier today to find other parents of multiples in most parts of the country as well as online.

The expert view

Caroline Rice, fertility coordinator, TAMBA (Twins and Multiple Births Association)

'I'd say when baby rests, you rest, when baby sleeps, you sleep. Housework can wait – and that's where your network of family or friends come in – maybe they could do the ironing for you or one of your friends could come and sit with the babies while you go into the kitchen and do dinner or something. A support network is essential. We are all very good at the stiff upper lip, but sometimes you do have to let your guard down and say, "It would be nice if we could have a cup of coffee sometime, or just go and have half an hour away from the home" because it can feel like a prison. Support is one of the biggest assets that anybody can have and that doesn't have to come from a family member – it can come from anybody. It can even come from somebody at the other end of a telephone or on a website where they can go on to the message board and say that they are having a really tough day – and someone will always email back.

continued

'I think a routine is essential. It makes a difference dealing with any baby, but it is doubly important with twins. It's getting them into that routine so that they will go for a certain number of hours before feeding again, because otherwise you just turn into a feeding machine. Another important thing for a mother is to have designated "me" time. It makes things seem easier to cope with if you have a bit of time out, and family and friends can help with this.

'One of the pieces of information I give to mothers is to say that it doesn't matter how hard life gets, you can't get these years back and that's why you have to enjoy them. Enjoy all those snuggles and all the little things that will happen, and every day you will notice something different – just remember they are unique.'

The early days

Most women who have had fertility problems have impossibly rosy ideas of what the early days with a new baby will be like, and the gap between the idealised dreams and the tiring realities can be huge. For parents of multiples the gap between expectation and actuality is often far, far greater. The mental image of two downy little heads sleeping side by side is all too often shattered by the exhausting reality of screaming babies and a never-ending round of feeding and nappy changing. A routine can really help with multiples, as it ensures that there is some regular time for you to sleep and to recuperate between feeding and changing.

Women who've found it hard to get pregnant sometimes doubt their abilities as mothers, and research has found that they are often less confident during the first year of parenthood than those who have conceived naturally. If you feel lacking in confidence and need help, don't imagine that you are not doing things properly. In order to be a really together mother of twins or triplets, you need to accept all the help you are offered. Don't be too proud and don't expect that you ought to be able to do everything yourself. Think carefully about what people could do that would be most useful when help is offered. People often assume that what would be helpful would be for them to cuddle your babies for a while, but it may be that what would be far more useful would be for them to sweep your kitchen floor or put on a load of washing. Don't be afraid to ask for the help that you really need.

Postnatal depression

You are at greater risk of postnatal depression if you have had twins or triplets. Lack of sleep and sheer exhaustion may be partly to blame, and it is often harder to get out and about in the early days with twins, which can make you feel lonely and isolated. Everyone assumes that you should be delighted that you finally have all that you have ever wanted, and that can make it even more difficult if you aren't able to admit that you are having a tough time. Parents of more than one baby sometimes feel that they aren't able to bond with their children properly, or to spend the time with them that they would have liked. Although these concerns are common to all parents of multiples, they may not have started out with the very high expectations of parenthood that are common to those who have waited to get pregnant, and they may not feel as disappointed if they are not enjoying every moment of their new lives. (See also Chapter 6 for more on postnatal depression.)

The expert view

Jane Denton, director, The Multiple Births Foundation

'I think there is this great focus on the pregnancy, and often not enough thought about what is going to happen when the babies are born. Our advice is to look at getting as much practical help as possible and not declining any. I think one of the real risks for both mothers and fathers is that you just become chronically exhausted if you are not careful, and there is this feeling that because there are two babies, both of you ought to be up looking after them all the time. If you haven't got any additional help we always suggest that you consider doing a shift overnight where one parent gets up for the first part and the second parent for the other part – in as far as it is possible to do so.

'In terms of getting out of the house for the mother, you can become really quite socially isolated and there is a much greater temptation to think that it is so much effort to get the babies ready to go out that you won't bother. One of the things we talk through with parents, if they are able to afford private help, is how to make what they can afford go as far as possible. Maternity

continued

nurses may be excellent in those first few days, but they are usually very expensive and it may be better to have some practical help during the day with aspects of coping at home – the washing, the shopping, the basic routine domestic chores – rather than somebody who is just focused on the baby.'

Living with multiples

However overwhelming it all seems at first, you will get used to your new family life, although it is true that there will be precious little spare time in the first few years. Looking after two or three babies can leave you feeling that you have no space or energy left for anything else in your life, but remember that it will get easier as your babies grow and are able to do more and more for themselves.

It is important even at an early age to ensure that your children are established as individuals, and this is particularly relevant for identical twins. Try to dress them differently, to let them have their own toys and belongings, to give them some time away from one another now and again and to call them by their names rather than always referring to them as 'the twins' or 'the triplets'. Encourage other people to do this too, as the children need to feel that they have their own identities.

It's easy to spend all your time thinking about your children, but don't forget your partner. Multiples can put a huge strain on your relationship. Life has changed from being just the two of you, able to do what you wanted, when you wanted, to being part of a family of four or more where you are both constantly on the go looking after the children and never have a spare moment. Make some time to spend together, however difficult this may feel. Plan ahead, book a babysitter and go out together now and again even if it's just for an hour or two. You need some time for yourselves as you both need to feel appreciated and listened to, and yet making time for one another often falls off the bottom of the to-do list. If you have an older child, make sure that they get some time alone with each of you too. An existing child often feels left out and neglected because of the amount of time two or three young babies can take up, and you may need to take it in turns to look after the babies now and then so that you can spend some one-to-one time with your older child.

Once you get into the swing of things and have a routine established for feeding your babies, things can get much easier, but when your babies start moving you will face a whole host of new challenges. You'll need to keep an eye on two or three children at the same time, which is hard work if they decide to head off in opposite directions. At home, a playpen can be helpful to contain the children safely, and when you are out you may need to use reins.

Your children's different characters will emerge more strongly as they get older, and it can be fascinating to watch as they grow and the dynamic between them changes. It is inevitable that you will make comparisons between them, but try to avoid letting them become too aware of this, as it can affect self-esteem if they compare themselves to a brighter or quicker sibling.

It is also important to allow them to develop their individuality, as this can prevent them becoming too dependent on one another. When they start school you may be asked to decide whether to put them in the same class, and this is something you will have to discuss as a family, as there are advantages and disadvantages. Friendship issues can be difficult for twins and there may be problems with jealousy once they start making their own friends. If your twins are non-identical and are not the same sex, it can be easier, but identical twins often have friends in common and may always be invited everywhere as a duo, which is sometimes difficult.

Once the children are ready for secondary school, it may be appropriate to send them to different schools. Academic comparisons are more obvious at this age, and the competition between twins can become more intense. As they enter the teenage years, the desire to separate from the family begins to grow, and with twins and triplets this includes separation from their sibling. It can cause problems if one is more mature and more ready to break the bond while the other is still quite dependent. At this age, one child may be more difficult, but try not to let them know that you feel they are the 'awkward one' as this can become a self-perpetuating problem!

For all the difficulties that can come with multiples, there are also many rewards. It is a challenge, but it is also an amazing experience for both you and your children. You will learn to become an incredibly efficient parent, it is also true that you won't have to go through the hassle and expense of fertility treatment in order to have more than one child, and your children will have a special bond for life that is unique.

Louise's story

Louise had a miscarriage after getting pregnant naturally, and she and her partner, Ian, were eventually told to try IVF, which worked the first time for them.

'The clinic made it clear that if you did become pregnant you had a one in two chance of twins because they put back two embryos. Because I was so pessimistic at that time, I had completely forgotten about it. I was totally bowled over to be expecting twins. I was genuinely very shocked that it had worked. Once I found out, we went for hormone-level tests and they were sky high, so the nurse said you may want to prepare yourself for multiples. Then on the scan, it revealed two babies.

'I was delighted because when you've lost a baby and you know you can't conceive naturally, you do think that even if one of these babies doesn't make it, we might have one child. I felt I had two chances of having a healthy child. We were absolutely delighted but incredibly anxious. In fact that went through the whole pregnancy. I was convinced that it wouldn't work again because I had lost a baby previously.

'I found the pregnancy a terribly difficult process. Every day was like a year – it was so long and so difficult because of losing a baby in the past and knowing that if we lost these babies we would be back to fertility treatment, not just trying again for another child.

'There were difficult times. Twin pregnancies are very complex and at about 12 weeks I went for a scan and was rather manhandled by the consultant who was doing the scan and after that I had a massive bleed and thought I was going to lose them. The babies caused me problems throughout the pregnancy, I was in and out of hospital for monitoring and for one or two-night overnight stays because of drops in blood pressure, feeling very strange, not feeling the babies move – there were all sorts of things.

'I found the whole thing very draining. When I gave birth, I was already completely exhausted. When IVF results in a multiple pregnancy, you don't have a normal pregnancy so you have the emotional trauma of the IVF and then the physical trauma of a multiple pregnancy. By the time you become a parent you are delighted, but really wiped out.

'Looking back, my memories of pregnancy are of anxiety and concern. I didn't enjoy it. Lots of things can go wrong with multiple pregnancies and I realise now, having heard the stories of others, that I was very lucky. I still think I'd do the same thing again though – if you can carry twins to the end, then you don't have to go through IVF again.

'I always wanted an elective Caesarean, because I know most twin births end up in an emergency Caesarean section, so I said I wanted a section from the start. Actually, by 36 weeks, the hospital was having me in every other day for a scan. At the last one I could hardly walk because I was so big – I'm only a small person, but I put on about 4 stone [25kg/56lb] carrying the children, and at 5ft 3in [1.6m] and 12½ stone [80kg/176lb], I shuffled in and the consultant said, 'You are 37 weeks, let's take them out now.'

'I wasn't well after the birth, so it was a bit of a blur.

One of the children went to special care because she was on the tiny side, so I only had one of them with me. I just drifted in and out of consciousness – I am not sure why. Then unfortunately because of the weight of the children on my spine, I slipped a disc. I came home and then ended up being rushed back into hospital. It was a very traumatic time, and we had no family around us, so that was very hard.

'I knew a lady who was a doula, and I employed her for three hours a week. I usually slept, but it was just something to hold on to and she was tremendous in terms of moral support. At six months she took me out with the girls in the pushchair to do some shopping – I hadn't dared to do it on my own before – and that was the moment where I felt I could move on my own and try to do it. Unfortunately, the problems with my back and neck persisted on and off throughout those six months, so I was debilitated by the experience.

'It was all a blur and I can't remember chunks of the first year, because when you are feeding every three hours through the night with two babies, you are not just putting one baby back, you are settling two. Will they both go back to sleep? Will one be difficult? You just never know, and you can't count on getting any sleep ever, so you just have to catch it when you can. It's a massive shock to the system because you have to do everything twice, and mentally that's quite a leap to make. Once you expect it, you just do it and never think about it again, but it takes a while to reconcile yourself to the hard work involved.

'The baby stage was easier in terms of time for myself

because they would be in a cot and not moving around, and I would be able to lie on the bed and get some sleep, or at least have a shower, but it's very difficult once they start moving. With twins you are never alone, but you get used to that and it is a wonderful adventure, but it's all consuming, even now they are two and a half. They are very active and full of fun. It has become the most amazing, joyful thing, but what I always say to people expecting twins is, "Just hang on in there till about 18 months and then it changes." It took about that long to feel that you were getting a bit of your life back, that you were in control. People say twins are "double trouble", but it's almost like having two and a half children, because you have this added dimension of how they interact with each other, so it's not just double the workload, it's the dynamic between them that creates a problem.

'It is expensive in the beginning. I couldn't breastfeed, so all the milk had to be bought and all the nappies. It is very costly and there is no recognition of that for those of us with multiples. Also, often it just is not possible to pay for childcare if you have a part-time job. I am lucky, as I had a good job that allowed me to make it financially viable to put them into a private nursery, work three days a week and get some money – although not very much! At least I keep my foot in the door at work, which is why I have done it.

'My partner and I met as university sweethearts but having twins nearly destroyed us after 17 years together. I was so exhausted and then you become very bad tempered, and he just didn't help me. Some nights I would get up 20–25 times. You can't really explain it to people, because it sounds as if you are lying, but my girls were not good sleepers and so that was just absolutely debilitating.

'I felt this huge plummet, because you want this so much, and then when you get it, it's like being hit by a train. You do need a support network. If you can line it up beforehand that is very good. There is this mummy brigade of professional mothers where everything has to be organic and blended at home – just forget all that as a multiple mother. If you can go to a twins group before you have the babies, those women will throw their arms round you and try to help you – and they are the only people who can prepare you.'

CHAPTER 11

Donor Families

There are more than 2,000 children born every year in the UK alone using donor eggs and sperm, and donor conception has become part of everyday life. It may have been going on for decades, but in the past there was a real stigma attached to the use of donor sperm and it wasn't something that people talked about openly. Children were rarely told about their origins if they had been conceived using donor sperm. Now, we are far more open about the whole idea of donor conception and it has not only become much more common but it has also become a huge international business with people travelling from one country to another, as shortages of eggs and sperm and differing rules and regulations about eligibility and anonymity have altered the face of assisted conception.

No one starts trying for a child hoping that they will have fertility treatment, and you probably wouldn't choose to use donor eggs and sperm if you didn't have to, but donor conception has allowed many people to have families of their own who wouldn't otherwise have been able to. It can take a while to come to terms with the idea that you won't have your own genetic child, and people sometimes start out by assuming that they are having to accept a form of treatment which they feel is somehow 'second-best', because it wouldn't have been the way they had intended to have their children. There may always be an underlying sadness about the fact that you weren't able to use your own eggs or sperm, but once you have your family, this tends to be completely over-taken by the joy that being a parent can bring.

Anxieties about having used donor eggs or sperm often surface during pregnancy and right through to the early days after the birth, and it is perfectly normal to feel this way. For most people, any kind of anxiety is short-lived. It's not that you forget that your child was donor-conceived, but it just becomes part of your family's story. It was really summed up by a woman I interviewed who had used a donor egg to have her son; she explained, 'I don't ever think now that I wish my son had been from my eggs because it wouldn't have been him, and it feels so much like he was meant to be.'

Pregnancy after donor conception

As with any pregnancy after fertility problems, the initial euphoria at your success is often quickly accompanied by feelings of anxiety and concern. You are accustomed to dealing with the aftermath of month after month of trying to conceive unsuccessfully, and this is uncharted territory. The natural apprehension any prospective parent experiences is often exacerbated by concerns about the way you have had to get pregnant.

When you are dealing with infertility, the focus is tightly centred on getting pregnant and there is often little thought to what might happen once you succeed. People often progress quite rapidly down the path from trying to get pregnant naturally to trying to get pregnant with assisted conception, to using donor gametes. There is not always time to take a step back or the space to think and discuss things in depth. Of course, anyone using donor gametes is advised to have counselling before starting treatment, and the aim of this is to help iron out some of the anxieties that can arise during pregnancy and in the early days of parenting. Generally, this will be some kind of 'implications counselling' to ensure you have thought through the pros and cons of the path you are taking, and are fully aware of the consequences for your family. Unfortunately, in some cases, the implications counselling can become little more than a rubber-stamping exercise in order to get the go-ahead to start treatment. Most people only have one session, and there isn't always the opportunity to explore any inner concerns in sufficient depth, but there is no reason why you shouldn't have more counselling once you are pregnant, if it would be beneficial. Alternatively, talking to other people who have had their children after donor conception can be incredibly helpful as they will understand exactly how you may be feeling. You can find details of support networks at the end of the book.

The expert view

Mollie Graneek, specialist fertility counsellor

'I think people underestimate the need for counselling beforehand when they are using donor gametes. You are given this preliminary counselling session, but it is truly not enough. I think sometimes they do need more counselling even during pregnancy. The thing that comes up time and time again is that women are terrified that their baby is going to be ugly, although they don't want to voice it because it seems dismissive and shallow. They worry about what the baby will look like and whether they will be able to identify or bond with the baby. I think that what happens is that this fear becomes heightened – almost to a point where they start to imagine all sorts of disfigurement and things like that.'

Dealing with any worries and concerns

Some people feel that they have really prepared themselves for all eventualities and have addressed their worries and concerns in the time leading up to treatment. Whether you have used donor sperm, donor eggs or both, the tiny cells that are now growing are being nurtured by your body, and being pregnant, watching your body change and feeling the baby moving, are all an integral part of the process of bonding with your baby. Most women find that they feel closer to their baby as the pregnancy progresses and that any concerns are gradually assuaged during these nine months.

However, anxieties that you couldn't have anticipated may arise. If you know next to nothing about the donor, or have only limited information, this can raise questions and concerns about what your child will be like. There are no conclusions to the age-old debate as to whether children are shaped by nature or nurture, whether it is their genes or their upbringing that makes them the people they become, but we know that a child's environment plays a huge role in establishing his personality and behaviour. It is very common to worry about the baby's appearance, because you haven't usually seen the donor. Women do sometimes get quite focused on this and start to imagine that they might not be able to bond with their baby because it will look peculiar or unattractive or have some kind of weird features or deformity. Many women have these concerns, but often find it hard to admit to them. Remember that really most babies look very similar and there is absolutely no reason for your baby to be any different. I have talked to dozens of women who have worried about what their donor-conceived baby might look like during their pregnancy but not one who has thought that their baby was in any way unattractive once it was born.

Prospective parents may also worry that their child will have an unequal relationship with them, being closer to the genetic parent. In fact, all the evidence shows that this is not the case at all in donor families, and the children's relationships with the non-genetic parent are just as good if not even better. People often try to bottle these feelings up, refusing to acknowledge them because they can feel too huge and too fundamental to handle. Remember that it is far better to try to address your concerns before the baby comes along, and you may find it really helpful to talk to others who have conceived using donor gametes.

In some countries, you can now access donor treatment within a matter of weeks, which is often very welcome for anyone who has spent years struggling to get pregnant, but can have unexpected disadvantages if there isn't time to think through all of the consequences. Fertility treatment can take on a momentum of its own and there may not always be sufficient time and space to think about how you will feel and how you will deal with things in the future. It's not to say that you wouldn't make the same decisions if you had time to think about them, but just that you might be better prepared for any doubts and concerns that you may feel further down the line. You may not be offered any counselling before donor treatment if you are travelling overseas, but it is not too late to seek this out at any stage of pregnancy or parenting.

There is no reason for your pregnancy or the birth to be different because you have used donor eggs or sperm, and I have come across people who've had treatment overseas who have decided not to tell their doctor or midwife about their treatment because they feel this is a purely personal issue and of no relevance to anyone else. It is important to be honest, however, because there can be some consequences. If you have used a donor egg, your age-related risk of chromosomal problems may be far lower than would normally be expected, as egg donors are usually younger than recipients. The risk assessments you will be given in any antenatal testing will not be accurate unless you have been truthful. There are also some increased risks during pregnancy for women who have used donated eggs; for example, there is a greater chance of getting pre-eclampsia, and your doctor or midwife won't be aware that you are at higher risk if you have not told them about your treatment.

The expert view
Olivia Montuschi, Donor Conception Network

'It can be quite common for people to panic when they are pregnant. I think a lot of the worries are ones to do with just not trusting your body, and I think this happens with ordinary IVF pregnancies and not just donor pregnancies – you have lost faith in your body and suddenly you are pregnant and you've lost faith in your ability to sustain this pregnancy and for things to be OK. The more attempts you've had, the more odd and unusual you have come to feel, the less you trust your body to work normally. I do come across anxieties about bonding but they are not as great as you expect, particularly for women, because once you are pregnant you feel so right and just so connected to the baby. I can think of cases where women have had great difficulty in bonding, but my sense is that these are people who may have had bonding difficulties anyway.'

Birth after donor conception

When it comes to the birth itself, parents of donor-conceived children are sometimes concerned about the initial moment of bonding, and worry about how they may feel when they first see their child. If you don't know what the donor looks like, this is a perfectly natural concern. For any parent who has taken a long time to conceive, whether they have used donor gametes or not, there can be issues around the expectation of what you have imagined as the perfect moment of bonding with your baby after the birth and the reality of being presented with a crying baby when you are still feeling traumatised by the experience of labour. For some people it is a beautiful moment, but for many others it takes time for them to fall in love with their child. If you've used donor eggs or sperm you may immediately assume that the donor treatment is the cause of this, but it's far more likely to be related to the shock of being a new parent. Most people feel this and can find it overwhelming, no matter how they conceived their child.

The early days

Finding yourself at home with a newborn baby is hard work, and it's unfamiliar territory to most new parents. The idea that we have some instant inherited parental instinct that kicks in the moment we are faced with our own newborn baby just isn't true for most people, and everyone feels they are completely at sea at first. If your baby is donor-conceived, you may worry that this has some relevance when it comes to the difficulties you feel, but again, it is unlikely to have anything to do with whether or not you are genetically related to your child.

There may be some underlying feelings of sadness, anger or jealousy in the early days. Don't brush these under the carpet and try to forget about them. If you can talk about your feelings to your partner, or to a friend or a counsellor, accepting that they are a completely normal reaction, it will be far easier to move on. As you become more accustomed to family life, the way in which your child was conceived will gradually fade into the background.

Christopher's story

Christopher and his wife, Judy, have twins born as a result of IVF using donor sperm. He feels he hadn't dealt with the consequences of this emotionally before they had treatment.

'Logically and rationally my head was saying that this was the only option and I didn't have a problem with it — it was either that or we didn't have children. It comes across as a bit of a no-brainer when you weigh it up like that. I put to one side the fact that I was never going to have children of my "own" and I thought I would come back and deal with it later. The counselling we had didn't involve the impact of my infertility on our lives at all. It was only after my wife was pregnant that we then realised that there were issues we needed to deal with.

'Despite the fact that having the children was something

that we were doing together, for me it was quite a lonely experience and I felt that there was quite a lot that my wife didn't really understand. She thought that once we had the children that was pretty much it. I believed it because I wanted to believe it, and it seemed wrong, when we had waited for so long, for me to throw a spanner in the works. Everyone expects that when the babies come along it is all going to be fine, but it's a very stressful experience.

'I know that a lot of guys are concerned about how they will feel. The best way for me to describe it is that it is quite something to face up to the fact that, ultimately, I am a genetic cul-de-sac; for me to think that genetically I am a dead end is a profound thing. It makes you ask questions about what you are here for. How do I leave my mark on the world? How do I balance the emotional impact of this genetic dead-end thing with the two beautiful children that I have at home? They have no other father than me and I want to be a father to them. In many ways it affects my relationship in a positive way, as I try harder to be there for them and give them more attention. One of the things that has really concerned me is what happens if I am not here any more? What connection do they have to me if I were not here? One of them in particular is so very, very like me and I can see the impact that I have on them, but nevertheless the question is still there in my mind all the time.

'My wife assumed that because I said donor treatment seemed like a good idea, that meant that I had dealt with everything that there was to deal with. The aim was to have a family, and we got our family, but we are still dealing with the fallout of that now. By the time you get to the point where you realise that something is wrong, you want to press ahead, and the last thing you want to do is say, "Let's just put this on hold" while you go over all your issues, but I really would say to people that it's worth it. If I had my time again now, I would have slowed it down. Taking the time to assess what it means to you and your life and what life is going to be like when the child comes along has got to be worth doing.'

Should you tell your children about their conception?

Families have been created using donor sperm for decades. In fact, the first recorded case was in 1884 when a woman who was unable to get pregnant with her husband was inseminated with donor sperm by a doctor while she was sedated. The doctor who carried out the insemination had been unable to discover any reason why the woman and her husband were unable to conceive and eventually decided to try to achieve a pregnancy using sperm donated by one of his medical students. The doctor didn't see fit to tell the woman, who gave birth nine months later, what he had done, although her husband was later informed and asked for it to be kept secret from his wife. It was a huge step forward medically, but at the same time established an aura of shame and secrecy around the procedure that it has taken a long time to shake off. Nowadays, parents who have used donor eggs or sperm tend to be more open, but there are still some who feel they would rather not tell their children the truth; perhaps because they want to protect them from what they feel themselves to be a stigma or because they are worried that telling them will spoil close family relationships. Sometimes it comes down to the simple fact that they just don't know how to broach the subject with their children.

If you feel you don't want your children to know, you need to think carefully about your motives for this and about the possibility that they may discover the truth at some point in the future. It is very difficult to keep a secret within a family, and your child or children may well sense that there is something they don't know or are not being told. Some people may find it easier than others to deal with secrecy and the white lies that it can entail, but it can be incredibly stressful to be on your guard all the time, constantly watching yourself so that you don't let anything slip. It can also lead to a sense of guilt and shame about the donor conception, which would not be there otherwise. If you have told any other family members or friends that you have used donor gametes, there is a high risk that this may emerge at some point in the future and that your child will discover the truth in a way that is far from ideal. You need to be very clear about this if you have decided you don't want to tell, and to be sure that you can prevent your child from ever finding out in unexpected circumstances. Unfortunately, even when parents have spent many years successfully avoiding telling their children about their conception, the truth does sometimes emerge, perhaps accidentally as the result of a family argument or after a parent has died. This can be incredibly difficult to deal with later in life.

The expert view

Olivia Montuschi, Donor Conception Network

'If there's anything you would want to have at the centre of family relationships it is trust, and not telling puts a lie at the heart of the family. Time and again we hear donor-conceived adults say that they became aware at some point that there was something odd in the family about them and wondered if they were adopted, or they have thought that perhaps their mother had had an affair with somebody. I do feel strongly that early telling is the key to good stuff happening in the family. Fundamentally, it's easier — holding a secret is hard.'

Won't telling our child have an effect on our family relationships?

It is true that there are donor-conceived adults who feel very angry and misunderstood and who believe that their conception has caused them huge problems for the rest of their lives. One familiar thread that runs through nearly all of their stories is that they didn't find out the truth until they were teenagers or adults, and that they had often discovered accidentally rather than by design. Finding out later in life does mean that people have to completely reassess everything that they have understood about themselves, and inevitably this can lead to anger and confusion and can have a devastating effect on family relationships.

People often worry that the parent who is not genetically related to the child will find it harder to establish a relationship if they tell the truth. In fact, this is a parental preoccupation which doesn't seem to cause problems for children. Children tend to accept things easily if they feel they have always known them, and they view the people who look after them as their parents. Research has shown that children who were told that they were donor conceived at an early age don't seem to have any issues with it, but it can be highly destructive if the truth only emerges later in life, when discovering that something so fundamental has been kept secret can shatter an individual's sense of self.

The expert view

Professor Susan Golombok, director, Centre for Family Research, University of Cambridge

'Parents are sometimes worried that telling would ruin their relationship with their child, particularly the relationship with the non-genetic parent, and that the child wouldn't love them so much. Of those parents who have told their children, not one has had a bad experience. They all wondered afterwards what they were so worried about. If children are told when they are little it seems to be fine, and the people who seem to be upset about finding out they were donor-conceived are those who either found out by accident or were told when they were well into adolescence or early adulthood.

'Those who were told when they were little

continued

generally accepted it in the way that adopted children do – it has always been part of their lives. Some of the children said they didn't remember being told, that they had just always known, and that seems to be the best way. They don't really understand it at first, but as they get older they can ask more questions. In general, it's those who are told later on who are much more shocked, angry and upset.'

How to tell

It is clear that the earlier you tell your child, the easier it is. People are often very anxious about telling children when they are very young, because they fear that they won't understand. There may also be concerns about your child telling other people outside the family's close circle of friends and family, and what the reaction to this may be. You do have to be prepared for this, but remember, your child is telling people because he or she feels no sense of shame about it. Children are often quite proud of the fact that their parents wanted them so much that they had to have help to make them, and they may see this as something that makes them very special. If you have overcome any anxieties you may feel about it, this will help your child to have the same positive attitude.

If you are thinking about how to tell an older child, you may worry about finding the right time and the right way to do it. Parents who haven't told their children sometimes have feelings of discomfort about it themselves, and the one really important thing is to try not to transmit this to your child, as children are astute at picking up on parental unease. The Donor Conception Network's *Telling and Talking* booklets will help you to talk to your child about this in the right way, and they are aimed at specific age groups.

The expert view
Olivia Montuschi, Donor Conception Network

'It's very easy if you just start chatting to your child when they are very young about how sometimes mummies and daddies need some help to make a baby. You can look in our *Telling and Talking* booklet – it gives examples of the language that we suggest people use and you just build up the story bit by bit: "It takes a seed from a daddy and an egg from a mummy to make a baby, and sadly mummy's eggs or daddy's seeds weren't working, so we needed some help, and a kind man or lady helped us to make you." Certainly, with younger children you don't need to talk about sex at all. People worry that somehow you are despoiling a child's innocence – but in fact what they are doing is taking adult anxieties and hang-ups into a child's world where a child just doesn't share them at all.'

The family unit

As your children grow older, they will have their own questions about donor conception, but it seems that the more parents have told them, the less of an issue this becomes. People often worry before they start treatment that their relationships with their child will be unbalanced if only one has a genetic link to the child and fear that the other parent may be left out of the family bond. Researchers have found that this isn't the case at all, and that donor families are actually closer than most other families. There may also be concerns that the child will be affected in some way, but again this really doesn't seem to be the case at all. Research shows that donor-conceived children are generally well-functioning, well-adjusted children, that both parents tend to be equally involved and that they have good relationships with their children.

Single women

The numbers of single women having donor treatment has been steadily rising in recent years, as women balance the possibility of leaving it too late to ever have children against the desire to wait until they are in the right relationship. Women often worry that their decision to go it alone may be selfish, and that it may make things difficult for their child in the future, but there is no evidence of this. We tend to hold up the traditional two-parent family as an ideal, but what really matters is the environment a child grows up in, and being in a happy single-parent family is far better than living in an unhappy two-parent family.

You do need a good support network, as going through pregnancy, birth and the early years of parenting by yourself can be very lonely and isolating. Accept any offers of help that you get, as there will be little time for yourself, and don't feel too proud to let friends and family do what they can. Single mothers tend to get a bad press, but this is often due to a stereotypical image of a single-parent family, which may have very little relevance to your daily life.

The expert view

Professor Susan Golombok, director, Centre for Family Research, University of Cambridge

'People have this image of single parents as teenage mums or women on very low incomes on the edge of poverty and living in dire economic circumstances. Of course, that's the reality for some women, but what's interesting about single women having children by choice is that they don't experience some of the negative factors that are associated with the problems with single-parent families. Generally, these are older women who have thought about it hard and planned it, they are often professional women or women on high incomes, women who do have a lot of social support, who haven't just been through a divorce or separation and had all the stress associated with that, the child isn't separated from a parent with whom they'd had a relationship, so all of these things that are associated with problems in some kinds of single-parent families are not there with single mothers by choice who go to a clinic and have donor insemination.'

Lesbian couples

Having a family using donor sperm is something many lesbian couples now consider, and women are more often turning to fertility clinics when they want a baby because it is safer to use sperm that has been properly screened. As with any donor-conceived child, there are no reasons for pregnancy or birth to be any different.

Any concerns that having two mothers and no father might have a psychological effect on the children seem to have been comprehensively ruled out by the research into these families, which shows that they are generally extremely well-functioning. The other main area of concern is often that the children of lesbian couples might be teased or bullied by their contemporaries which could lead to emotional problems, but attitudes have changed hugely in the last few decades, and lesbian families are generally very well accepted; however, this can depend on where you live, and it may be easier for the children of lesbian mothers to feel accepted in a cosmopolitan urban environment than in a small rural village.

Trying again

Once you've had a child and know the joy that a family can bring, you may feel that you'd like to try to have another as soon as you can. When you've used donor eggs or sperm, you may wish to try to have the same donor again, as this maintains the genetic link in the family. You may feel this would make you more of a family unit.

If you've had IVF and have any spare frozen embryos, that can seem a quick solution, but do keep in mind that the frozen embryo transfer may not always be successful just because the fresh cycle of treatment worked for you. You may then have to decide whether you want to try again using a different donor. Cost can sometimes be the deciding issue. Once you have a child, this rules out the possibility of funded treatment, and using donor sperm or eggs can be very expensive.

There are strict limits in the UK on the number of children that may be conceived using each individual donor's sperm. This is not such an issue for egg donors who often only donate once, but if you've used a sperm donor you may be asked up front to pay to store frozen sperm if you may want to use the same donor in the future. Sometimes this can be an expensive business, as a clinic may suggest that you should pay to keep all the donor's donated sperm frozen for your use until you've completed your family, at which point it can be released so that others could use it. Using the same egg donor can be more difficult as donating eggs is an invasive process and not something most women tend to go through many times. If you've been part of an egg-sharing scheme, the egg sharer may not be interested in another cycle, and may have got pregnant or had a child herself in the interim.

The expert view

Olivia Montuschi, Donor Conception Network

'A lot of people are desperate to have the same donor. I can understand that they feel that it is going to be important for the children to have full siblings and that somehow it makes them feel more of a proper family if the children all come from the same donor. Actually, there is a downside, because if you have two children from the same donor and they have very different attitudes to finding out information, you are really stuck. If one wants the information and the other doesn't, then the one searching compromises the other.'

Knowing more about the donor

In countries where donors are no longer anonymous, it will be possible for your child or children to find out more about the donor when they are older. In the UK, the law changed in 2005 and children born after the change in the law will be able to access identifying information once they reach the age of 18. They will be able to discover whether they were donor-conceived, whether they could be related to a potential partner and whether they have any donor-conceived siblings, as well as identifying information about the donor.

The expert view

Professor Susan Golombok, director, Centre for Family Research, University of Cambridge

'We've been looking at mothers of donor offspring who are searching for the donor and their donor siblings and what happens when they meet up. The children are much more interested in their donor siblings, their genetic half-siblings living in other families, than they are in their donor. They want to meet the donor, but they are much more interested in forming a relationship with their half-siblings in other families. In our studies we don't find much regret about having searched and found out. Some meet and make contact and don't carry on, but more often than not they do maintain contact and are pleased to do so.'

Not all donor-conceived adults want to find their donor, and when they do it is often out of curiosity more than anything else. It can feel slightly threatening to you as a parent, but finding the donor doesn't mean replacing you as a parent. For your child, you are his or her parent. The donor may have helped to conceive them, but being a parent means looking after your child and bringing them up, and this is a very different role. Your child may also want to find out about any half-siblings, and they can end up playing a bigger part in your child's life in the future, as it may be more easy to incorporate half-siblings into the extended family.

Amanda's story

Amanda and Dan had three cycles of IVF before egg donation was recommended.

'We had one cycle of egg sharing and I got pregnant on the first try, which was fairly amazing. I thought if I got pregnant I'd be hanging the flags out and running up and down the street, shouting and screaming, but actually I felt quite anxious because I had got used to accepting and dealing with failure, and to recovering from that. I'd got used to getting ready for bad news, and when it was good news I almost couldn't believe it. I was delighted and thrilled but I didn't quite know how to deal with it. The long journey had come to an end, but immediately I was worried about whether it was going to be OK.

'I struggled with the transition from IVF to egg donation, because it was like letting go of something, it was like a grieving process, because I was giving up this whole notion of having my own genetic child. I found that incredibly difficult and it took quite a while for me to accept that this was the route I was going to take and to feel at ease with it. I definitely felt as if I was jumping off one set of rails and onto another, and I found it very helpful talking to other mums who had had children through egg dona-tion. By the time I had treatment and was pregnant, I had dealt with a lot of the concerns I had early on about how I would feel. For me it immediately felt like *my* pregnancy, because it is all happening to you and that was very steadying for me, but I did find myself thinking, *What if I think this baby is really ugly when it is born; will I look at it and think it has got nothing to do with me?* I did have those concerns, but they weren't preoccupying thoughts. As the pregnancy went along it just felt more and more as if this was my child, and that whole process is really positive.

'I think, after the birth, I probably had the same worries as any other new mum, but I couldn't figure out whether it was just me being a new mum or whether it was me being an egg-donation new mum. I found quite a lot of comfort from talking to other mums who had normally conceived children, as a lot of the things that I was worrying about were also being reflected by them – things like worrying about whether I was bonding with my baby. I was very anxious in the first few months and I did feel over-whelmed by it. In my darkest moments, when we were exhausted and worried and I couldn't settle her, I did worry that maybe it was because she wasn't my genetic child. I know that is ridiculous and it has faded into the background now, but it was an extra layer of stuff that I felt I had to contend with. It wasn't the easiest of times for me, and I found myself thinking that I was not myself and was unrea-sonably anxious. It could just be because you are tired and it is so different from anything you have ever experienced – and it is really hard work as well. I would advise talking to other mums as much as possible and trying to reassure yourself that actually what you are experiencing is probably just new-mum worries and not necessarily because this isn't your genetic child. You do get things out of perspective in the early stages of parenthood.

'It just got easier and I got more confident and relaxed into it a bit more. At around a year my daughter was a lot more settled. I felt as if I knew the ropes and, gradually, this whole mad anxiety just faded away, things just seemed to get a lot easier. It is still in my mind. I do think about it quite often but it is not a negative thing, it is just completely part of my everyday life, it's my reality, part of the fabric of my life, and it couldn't be anything other than that. My daughter is donor-conceived and that is just how our family is.

'I have a little children's book about being donor-conceived and we started reading it to her when she was months old. We do talk about it and she really likes to hear the story so it's a nice way of starting to talk to her about it. I don't know anything about the donor. I'm comfortable with the situation, with the way that we've formed our family, but for me it has been better for it to be anonymous with the opportunity for my daughter to get information at a later stage. When, and if, she wants to do that I will be really interested, I'd love to meet the donor, but only if my daughter wants to meet her. I would like to say thank you.

'Even though it has been an unconventional route to motherhood, I am so thrilled and proud of my family. Any times of doubt and conflict have been vastly outweighed by the positive experience of raising my daughter, and I would do it all again in a heartbeat. Although technically speaking there are three people involved in making our daughter who she is, I feel 100 per cent her mum. She is absolutely my heart and soul, and I couldn't love her any more than I do.'

CHAPTER 12

The Teenage Years and Beyond

By the time our children are ready to leave primary school, most of us have adjusted to our role as parents and are feeling less pressured and more confident; however, our relationships with our children were formed around our experiences of infertility, and although the focus on that phase of our life may soften, it doesn't stop having an influence.

Although my own infertility is very much in my past and being a parent has become an integral part of who I am, I am still aware of how lucky I am to have my children. It seems to be a common thread among parents who had a struggle to have their children that we don't want to ever take our children for granted. The depth of feeling may be related to the intensity of the experience of trying to get pregnant in the first place, as someone who has been successful with their first attempt at fertility treatment will inevitably find it a less painful memory than someone who went through multiple treatment cycles or miscarriage, but we all have that same sense of gratitude. Most parents who struggled to conceive remain convinced that their experiences have altered them and continue to have an impact on the way they feel about their family and interact with their children.

The transition from childhood to the teenage years

The path to becoming a teenager is far from straightforward, and your child can seem to lurch between childhood and adulthood; one minute appearing astonishingly grown-up in her views and opinions, and the next behaving like a five year old. It can be a testing time for any parent, and it brings a whole set of new challenges as you try to work out how best to deal with your changing child. Try to remember that this is a steep learning curve for anyone and that most parents don't always feel confident that they are getting things right.

An integral part of this transitionary stage is the move from primary to secondary school. In the final years at primary school, your child has probably started to seem very mature compared to the tiny children in the early years' classes, and you will have grown used to seeing her in this way. It can come as a shock to realise that the bigger children in secondary school will be young adults, and your child will suddenly look very small and vulnerable in comparison. If you live in an area with a middle school system, these differences may not be quite so stark, but it is still a time of great change.

It can feel very sad to say goodbye to your child's primary school, and to the life you've grown used to. When you didn't have children, it was these early years that you probably yearned for; the bright blobby children's pictures on your walls, the toys and games, the summer fair and the school Nativity play, and you were unlikely to have had longing visions of a grumpy teenager slouching around the house. Knowing that you are leaving this stage of life behind you for good does feel sad, but the path ahead as you watch your child grow into an adult can be just as rewarding, albeit in a very different way.

Until this point, your child will have gained independence gradually, but when she moves to secondary school, she can seem to take giant steps almost overnight. For a parent who may still feel overprotective of a long-awaited child, this period of sudden change can be daunting. Up until now, you will have known the parents of your child's friends, you may have walked to school with her every day and popped in to see her teacher if any concerns arose. Suddenly, you can find that you don't know the first thing about any of her friends, she may be getting a bus or train to school by herself and she will have dozens of different teachers. The cosy existence you have grown comfortable with can feel as if it has been turned upside down. Although initially it may all be rather worrying, parents often find that their child surprises them by taking things in her stride with an unexpected level of maturity.

On my son's induction day at senior school, it was suggested that it was a good idea for parents not to do too many things for our children that they were capable of doing for themselves. It made me realise quite how much I did for my son that he was perfectly able to do himself; making his bed, cleaning his shoes, packing his school bag, reminding him to brush his teeth and to tidy his room. I decided to make a conscious effort to stop doing at least some of them and let him get on with it without interfering. I was worried that everything would descend into chaos, but I was amazed at how quickly he managed to do the things that mattered to him without any help from me; so he never forgets his rugby kit or football training, but mysteriously always manages to overlook the need to make his bed and clean his shoes!

Learning to let go

One of the difficult things about living with infertility is the loss of control, and as a parent of a young child you regain some of that control over not only your own life but also your child's. You make the decisions about what your child does and when, and the level of freedom that you choose to give him is a matter of individual parenting style. As your child grows older, and particularly after this transition to senior school, you will find that he starts to move further apart. It can be quite subtle at first, but gradually you will find that you don't always know exactly what he is doing or who he is with.

Having felt more in control of life for some years, the thought of having to let go again can seem rather unnerving, and most parents feel anxious about what lies ahead. There are bound to be conflicts and hiccups along the way, but it is important to remember that this separation is part of growing up. Letting your child go to school alone and allowing him to go out with friends to the park or to the cinema can seem an alarming prospect when you are accustomed to knowing exactly where he is all the time. Most parents sit and watch the clock the first time their child is out without any adults, and that's why it's so important to establish ground rules beforehand: make sure you know who your child is with and set an agreed time for him to return. Once he appreciates that following your rules will mean that you will trust him in future, this can all be less painful than you'd anticipated, and try to remember that it is part of your child's natural development to start to strike out alone.

Getting the right balance

Perhaps the most difficult challenge to helping your teenager negotiate her way through the transition to adulthood is managing to get the balance right between giving your child the freedom she needs in order to develop while continuing to offer the guidance and support that she will often require. Teenagers may be growing into young adults, but that doesn't mean that they don't need boundaries. Everyone has their own ideas about where these lie, and you may find that you are stricter than your child's friends' parents about certain things at the same time as being more relaxed about others. It can be hard to know when you need to step in and play the stern parent and when you should step back and allow your child to make her own mistakes. This is a learning process for the parent as much as for the child and one where rules are subject to constant renegotiation.

It can be tempting to keep stepping in to ensure that your child follows the right path, and although, of course, there are times when you need to intervene, there may be others when you will have to wait to be able to say, or at least think, 'I told you so'! Research has shown that parents who have children after fertility treatment tend to become close-knit family units, and this can really make a difference. As my own children have grown older, I've come to realise quite how much faith I have in them. It makes it easier to allow them to follow their own paths. Although I know things won't always run smoothly, it does help a lot if you have an underlying trust and confidence in your child.

The other thing to remember when you are dealing with a teenager is that your experiences of infertility may have left you with some strengths that you didn't realise you had. Living with fertility problems is tough and you will have established coping skills in order to get through the difficulties without necessarily being consciously aware of that. If you do encounter some thorny obstacles along the way, you may find that you deal with them far more ably than you would have expected.

Growing older in the face of a new generation

Of course, the other side of watching your children grow up is the knowledge that you are getting older too. Many of us came to parenthood later in life than we would have anticipated, and as we watch our children develop into young adults, our own lives are changing too. Our children's lives are opening up ahead of them as ours gradually start to slow down, and this can make you feel very middle-aged.

For women, this can be particularly difficult. When you've struggled to conceive, the menopause brings the emotional hurdle of accepting that the final miracle naturally conceived baby you may have occasionally allowed to drift into your subconscious is never going to arrive, and that the fertility that didn't come easily is now leaving for good. The phase leading up to the menopause, known as the peri-menopause, can go on for years, and during this time the majority of women do experience some symptoms, although they vary hugely from one woman to another. If you start reading up on menopausal symptoms it sounds a pretty ghastly experience with everything from hot flushes, thinning hair, weight gain and joint pain, as well as mood swings, depression, irritability and anxiety. Don't panic, as around a quarter of women don't experience any menopausal symptoms at all, and even those who do are unlikely to experience the whole lot at once. Whatever your symptoms, or lack of them, women who have thought they'd completely come to terms with their fertility problems can be surprised to find that they sometimes come back to haunt them at this time.

A young adult

If you think back to your own teenage and college years, life at this age is often full of the traumas of growing up. You can safely say that there will be a falling out, a broken heart and an alcohol-related incident of some kind along the way. While it's famously difficult for children to think of their parents as sexual beings, most parents have just the same difficulties with the idea of their children starting to have relationships and bringing home their first partners. It can be hard for us to accept that our precious babies are becoming fully fledged adults and that we can't always be there at their sides to protect them and care for them.

The empty-nest syndrome

After years of living with the day-to-day chaos of family life, the thought of your child spreading his wings and living elsewhere is not going to be easy, whether he's off to college, to work or to live with a partner. Some parents say that they relish their new-found freedom, but anyone who has struggled to have their child will probably feel that they'd rather continue to put up with the damp towels strewn across the bathroom floor, the piles of dirty washing and the fridge that magically empties just hours after being replenished. Having longed for a family for so long, it can seem as if the whole experience has flashed past without time to truly relish every moment of it. Perhaps it may be some consolation that nowadays children often return to live with their parents again after college, and that this may not be a final departure. There will be new pleasures from your relationship with your offspring that you may never have anticipated, and this doesn't signal the end of being a parent, but rather the start of being a parent to an adult rather than a child.

Susan's story

Susan and Jim had been through eight cycles of IUI when Susan got pregnant naturally after a holiday. They lost their baby when Susan miscarried at 20 weeks. They conceived Scott, now 14, after their first IVF cycle. Scott was born at just 26 weeks, and spent the first nine and a half weeks of his life in hospital.

'Everything revolved around Scott when he was a baby. I was never one for leaving him with anybody and used the excuse that I was breastfeeding and couldn't leave him. I took the decision that there was no way that I was going back to work after waiting for so long to become a mum. I fitted in with him rather than making him fit in with me. He was always a baby who needed his sleep and was in bed at seven o'clock, so we never went anywhere in the evenings for a long time because I wouldn't interrupt his routine. I just felt that he was the most important thing, and to be honest he probably still is the most important thing. I would put him first before anything else.

'We had six frozen embryos left after Scott was born and tried them two at a time. Each time one survived and one didn't, and we had it replaced but it never happened. At that point, having lost one baby and then gone into early labour and had a premature baby, we probably shouldn't have even tried again, but I really wanted another baby and I couldn't take the decision not to use the frozen embryos. When that didn't work I accepted that it just wasn't meant to be. I am happy now with what we have, although it took a few years to actually accept that we were only going to have one child, and I am very conscious of the fact that we never managed to complete our family.

'I never doubted my parenting skills and I was never fazed by being a mum, even though Scott was so small when we brought him home. You couldn't put him in his pram because he was too small, and if you put him in his crib you couldn't hear him cry if you weren't right beside him. He mewed like a kitten for the first couple of weeks. I just felt that we had tried so hard and now we actually had this baby, it was all going to be all right. Parenting seemed to come naturally, but I put pressure on myself to be the best parent that I could be.

'There is this obligation to be a superparent, when actually you are just a parent the same as anybody else – you are entitled to get cross and tired and fractious and have a normal relationship with your children, but you don't feel that you can allow yourself to do that. I always felt that having tried for so long to be a mum and to have a baby, it all had to be perfect. You put so much pressure on yourself, or at least I did, to be this perfect mum. I think because you have thought about it for so long, you have this rose-tinted vision of what motherhood and family life will be like. Everything has been coloured by the fact that you think it will be perfect because it is what you wanted, but it doesn't always work out that way. It probably took until almost the end of primary school before I stepped back a little bit and accepted that actually I didn't have to be this perfect superparent, that I was doing quite a reasonable job and I didn't have to put a lot of pressure on myself.

'The one thing I've always said is that infertility never leaves you, no matter what the outcome is, whether you are successful or not. Even having been successful, it is still always there and I still look at women in supermarkets shouting at their kids and think that they shouldn't be talking to them like that – children are special, they are precious. I still feel that a lot of people take their children for granted and if they just knew how special they were and how some people struggle, then perhaps they might be different.

'Scott still feels very precious, very special and I still look at him and think how lucky we are to have him, but I don't think I put the same pressure on myself any more. It was probably just after we got over the hurdle of the move from primary to secondary school and he was settling down and didn't have any problems – it was about then that I accepted that what I was doing was probably OK.

'I think we are still very close. Although he's grown up in some ways, he's still very cuddly, he still shares everything with me and we still talk about everything. He does have his own private life but it's not a huge part of what he does. When he's in the house, we're interacting all the time – if he's on the computer and I am on the computer, we're chatting and I share things with him, he helps me when I am stuck with all the techie stuff and he's quite happy to do that. I don't feel yet that he has gone off on his own and left me behind, but that might come.

'If we hadn't gone through what we went through, I don't think that we would have been as close. I think it does shape you and it shapes the way you bring your children up and therefore the way that they interact with you. He knows he is very special, not because he was IVF-conceived but because we struggled for so long – the issue for us has always been that we tried so hard for so long, that we lost one baby and almost lost Scott and that makes him extra-special rather than the fact that we needed IVF.

'It's the struggle and the time and effort that goes into it that just makes you appreciate how special your children really are. Every baby is precious, every one is special, but when you have had such a struggle to get there, they are even more precious. Even though Scott is 14, I still look at him and think how lucky I am. I think people who haven't had that struggle tend to take their children for granted. I don't mean that in a bad way. It's just that if anything comes easily to you, you don't appreciate it as much.

'The experiences you have before you have your children really shape the relationship that you have with them. Although I would never want anybody to go through what we went through, I actually wouldn't change what happened. I was totally distraught when we lost the baby and it still hurts now when I talk about it, although it was 16 years ago, but I wouldn't change it because I feel it has made me the parent that I am. It has made a difference to the person I am, and I think it has made me a better person, not just as a mum.'

Being a long-awaited 'baby'

I was interested in talking to some of the children, or young adults, who had been conceived after their parents had experienced fertility problems and exploring whether they thought it had made any difference to their lives. For those now in their twenties, being an IVF baby had been more unusual. In 1985, there were just 513 IVF babies born in the UK so it would have been quite something to be conceived that way. Even as relatively recently as 1995 there were only 5,791 IVF babies, while more recent statistics put the current figure at more than 15,000 each year. The children born in the earlier days of fertility treatment inevitably felt more special, and the fact that they are now older has given them an additional insight into infertility and treatment. For the majority of younger teenagers and children, the way in which they had been conceived seemed to feel totally irrelevant. I did, however, hear anecdotally that some were secretly rather pleased that they hadn't had to live with the unmentionable idea of their parents having intercourse in order to conceive them!

Infertility may have had a huge impact on your life, and fertility treatment may have transformed your future by giving you the child you longed for, but for those children themselves any sense of stigma has long disappeared. They may feel grateful for the technology that allowed them to be here, but it certainly doesn't seem to cause them any worries or concerns.

The expert view

Professor Susan Golombok, director, Centre for Family Research, University of Cambridge

'When we went back at 18 to the children conceived by IVF and interviewed them, IVF was such a non-issue for them. Some of them said they'd actually forgotten all about it until we'd gone to interview them. Being conceived by IVF from the children's point of view is just really not very interesting. We didn't get an impression that anyone was at all bothered by it.'

Talking to children and young people who had been conceived after their parents had experienced fertility problems and had been through treatment was fascinating for me. The infertility, which had been a source of so much pain and anguish, had ceased to have any negative impact when it came to the children. Being an IVF baby might sometimes bring a sense of pride, but for most of them it played a minor background part in their lives and certainly wasn't a source of anxiety or embarrassment.

'I don't ever think about being an IVF baby. It doesn't make me any different, and I don't think it makes my family different either. I don't feel the need to tell people about it because there is no point. When we covered assisted conception at school, I told the whole class that I was an IVF baby – I don't worry about telling people if it comes up. One boy in my class called me a tube baby as a joke, and the teacher got all worried that I might be really upset about it. Actually, I thought it was weird that she was worried because I couldn't see that there was anything to be upset about.

'Sometimes at primary school, if people knew they used to ask me if I'd been modified and whether I had any kind of superpowers. People still ask things like that occasionally, but now most of them are joking – although some of them really do think that's what happens!'   *Alfie, 14*

'I understand what my parents went through to have me and know that it makes a big difference to them. I know that I am very special to them and they think about me a lot differently than they would if they hadn't gone through all that. I obviously can't compare my family with another family, but I would say we are very close.'   *Scott, 14*

'When I told one of my friends I'd been an IVF baby, she thought I'd actually been grown in a test tube. I suppose that's what people think if they hear about "test-tube babies". I don't often tell people, because it's not something that I ever think about really. I do know it helped my mum and dad though, and I know they really wanted me.'
          Emily, 17

'It doesn't make any difference to me being an IVF baby because I'm really just the same as all my friends. I do sometimes think about what would have happened if there wasn't IVF, because my parents wouldn't have been able to have me and I wouldn't be here. They would have had to adopt babies or something and it might have been sad for them. A few of my friends know, but I'd only tell them if we were talking about people not being able to have babies, because it's really not very interesting to anyone else.'   *Flora, 10*

'I think I did grow up feeling I was special, partly because my parents always told me I was. I always knew about the IVF and I don't remember anyone sitting me down and telling me – it's part of who I am. I'm an only child, and I know my parents would have liked more children because they'd always wanted a big family. As it was, I got all the attention and, although sometimes I used to envy people who had lots of brothers and sisters, there are definitely advantages to being the only one too. I'm proud of being an IVF baby and I do tell people. Most of them find it quite cool, although sometimes someone says something really stupid – they're usually the people you wouldn't want to spend time getting to know better anyway.'   *Lucy, 21*

'Mum and dad couldn't have babies, as mum had endometriosis and was unable to conceive naturally. So they looked into IVF and I was born in 1991. Three years later, they also conceived my little sister. We are both happy and reasonably healthy, but mum and dad decided not to have any more kids, as they thought they would only be able to have me, not expecting to be able to conceive my sister! I think IVF is fantastic, but it does annoy me that some people, for some ridiculous reason, do treat me differently because of it; for example, my old head of year when I was in sixth-form college, asked me if I would change colour if he prodded me because I was a test-tube baby. This really annoyed me because it doesn't mean I'm any different, just because I was made a different way! I am proud to be an IVF baby and always will be!'   *Daisy, 19*

'I was one of three fertilised eggs, two of which survived – me and my sister, Georgina. We saw Professor Robert Winston and we joke, because of our similar dark features, that he is our "Daddy"! We have pictures of us with him at his 1,000 babies celebration party, when were about two. I actually contacted him recently, and he said he would meet me and my sister and take us on a tour of the House of Lords and have a cup of tea with us! We haven't heard from him since but the offer was very kind anyway. I also joined the Facebook group, "Proud to be an IVF baby", and was in contact with Professor Winston's first ever baby – she invited me to come to her house to watch football! It's nice to be a part of the group.

'I do not remember a moment when I first knew or was told I was an IVF baby. I always remember knowing, which I think can only be a good thing really. I have never seen it as a big deal, but then perhaps that would be different if it had been hidden and thus made into a bigger deal, I'm not sure. I never remember feeling strange about it, but not special either really. It was just accepted. A few friends used to call me Pinocchio – because I'm not a "real boy". It was all very good humoured. Nothing like that would ever be taken seriously, or said seriously because, I suppose, it was very obvious to me and my friends that there was nothing controversial or wrong with any of it.

'I think it is cool and can be a nice thing to tell people. We joke that me and my twin were "buy one, get one free", as the cost of the treatment would obviously be the same however many eggs were successful. She was first out by six minutes and thus I was the freebie! I have told friends I was a test-tube baby, and often it's one of the first things I tell people. They usually react very well. I've never had a negative reaction, actually. Most are interested and ask questions.

'I think it is funny that we have a price tag on us – that is a slightly strange feeling. I always feel extraordinarily grateful for life and for everything we have, and recently I have felt very grateful toward my grandmother because I learnt that she had paid the money for the IVF. I never thought until recently about the actual process of it all, when I realised it was a bit strange not to be conceived naturally. I also only just learnt about how it is actually done and that I was in a petri dish rather than a test tube. It certainly made an incredible difference to mum's life to have us. We are a very good unit together. Mum does always joke, however, about the fact that one easy mistake in the labelling of the dish and we might have been someone else's kids. I assume she's joking, but it's a valid point!

'I think perhaps we are all closer because of it. Mum, Georgina and I are very close, and me and my sister under-stand the sacrifices. Mum and Dad tried for seven years to conceive us. I try extremely hard with everything I do to give as much as I can to my family and to everyone around me. Thus I find it beyond crazy, I mean I think it is just madness, that "religious" people indulge in often utterly thoughtless argu-ment about the moral rights and wrongs of IVF.

'I am not sure if perceptions of IVF have changed. I am in southern America, playing tennis and going to university, and here there are an awful lot of conservative views around, so perhaps if I got into it with people here then the conversation would take a different course from how it would in England. Overall, IVF is an amazing thing which has given me and my sister two successful and happy lives so far, and made our mother very happy too, I think.'

Sam, 20

A future generation

One niggling concern for many parents who've experienced fertility problems is that their own children may find that they face similar challenges when they want to have families of their own. There is no evidence that this is the case, and the first ever IVF baby, Louise Brown, is now a mother herself along with many other adults conceived by fertility treatment. There have in the past been some questions raised about ICSI and whether the male fertility problems it overcomes might be passed on, but there is no clear evidence. While no one would like to see their children going through the pain of infertility, we may perhaps feel slightly reassured that developments in fertility treatment are moving forwards at a rapid pace, and that should our own children experience difficulties conceiving in the future, they are likely to be able to overcome them far more easily than we did.

Your future

The one thing that will almost definitely have been altered by your long journey to parenthood is yourself. No one goes through infertility and treatment without having been changed in some way. The degree to which you are affected may depend on your experiences, but your infertility will never leave you completely unscathed.

Some people feel that they have been left with a bitterness and anger that they can't quite get rid of, and may still feel jealousy and resentment towards others who are pregnant. This will usually fade, and in the longer term, most people seem to feel that their experience of infertility has changed them for the better, that they have perhaps become kinder, more empathetic and thoughtful people because of what has happened to them.

As you can see from the quotes above, the young people I spoke to for this chapter were, without exception, very grounded individuals, the sort of people who you instinctively felt would make a positive contribution to our society. Talking to them made me wonder whether our infertility could have a more positive legacy than we might ever have expected. Our children are growing up knowing that they were very much wanted and that they are loved and cherished. As parents we have been very concerned about trying to do the right thing for our children, and most of those who struggled to conceive seem to manage to avoid the trap of letting these much-loved children turn into the spoilt individuals others might expect them to be. Maybe the pain and trauma of our infertility wasn't in vain, maybe it has helped us to become the parents of a positive new generation of young people who will help to make the world a better place in the future.

Glossary

Amniocentesis A test carried out during pregnancy where a sample of amniotic fluid is taken to check for abnormalities.

Back-to-back (posterior) position This happens when a baby is lying facing outwards in the womb, with the back of the head pressing against the mother's pelvis.

Blastocyst An embryo which has been developing for about five days since conception.

CVS (chorionic villus sampling) A screening test carried out during pregnancy where a sample of tissue is taken from the placenta to check for abnormalities.

Doula Someone who provides non-medical support during labour and after childbirth.

Ectopic pregnancy An ectopic pregnancy occurs when a fertilised egg implants outside the womb, usually in the Fallopian tubes. It will not lead to a viable pregnancy.

Embryo A fertilised egg.

Gamete A sperm or egg.

HCG (human chorionic gonadotropin) A hormone produced during pregnancy that is measured in pregnancy testing.

ICSI (intra-cytoplasmic sperm injection) A variation of IVF during which sperm is injected into the egg to try to fertilise it.

IUI (intra-uterine insemination) A form of assisted conception where sperm is inserted into the womb.

Resources

United Kingdom

General

ACeBabes (offers support and advice to those who have families after assisted conception):
www.acebabes.co.uk

Infertility Network UK:
www.infertilitynetworkuk.com

NHS Direct (for health advice and reassurance):
www.nhsdirect.nhs.uk

Precious Babies (information about pregnancy, birth and parenting after infertility):
www.preciousbabies.org.uk

Pregnancy

National Childbirth Trust (NCT – offers support during pregnancy, birth and early parenthood): www.nctpregnancyandbabycare.org/home

Antenatal Results and Choices (provides support and information before, during and after prenatal testing): www.arc-uk.org

Birth

Association of Radical Midwives (midwives working to improve maternity care): www.midwifery.org.uk

Birth Trauma Association (supports women who have had a traumatic birth experience): www.birthtraumaassociation.org.uk

Bliss (special-care baby charity providing support and care for premature or sick babies): www.bliss.org.uk

Doula UK (non-profit organisation for doulas): http://doula.org.uk/

Independent Midwives UK: www.independentmidwives.org.uk

Miscarriage

The Miscarriage Association (support and information

for those suffering the effects of pregnancy loss):
www.miscarriageassociation.org.uk

SANDS (stillbirth and neonatal-death charity supporting
anyone affected by the loss of a baby):
www.uk-sands.org

Ectopic Pregnancy Trust (information, education and
support for those affected by ectopic pregnancy and those
caring for them):
www.ectopic.org.uk

Twins and multiple birth
TAMBA (Twins and Multiple Births Association):
www.tamba.org.uk

The Multiple Births Foundation:
www.multiplebirths.org.uk

Donor families
Donor Conception Network (self-help network for
families who have used donor gametes and for those who
are considering doing so):
www.donor-conception-network.org

Breastfeeding
La Leche League (breastfeeding support):
www.laleche.org.uk

The Breastfeeding Network:
www.breastfeedingnetwork.org.uk

Parenting

Contented Baby (for parents who follow routines):
www.contentedbaby.com

Daycare Trust (national childcare charity):
www.daycaretrust.org.uk

Family Lives (parenting advice and support):
http://familylives.org.uk

Mumsnet (online meeting point for parents):
www.mumsnet.com

Netmums (advice, information and support for mothers):
www.netmums.com

Pink Parents (for lesbian, gay and bisexual parents):
www.pinkparents.org.uk

Working Families (support for working parents and carers):
www.workingfamilies.org.uk

Older mothers

Mothers 35 plus (support for older mothers):
www.mothers35plus.co.uk

Problems

Association for Post-natal Illness (offers support and information):
http://apni.org/

Cry-sis (support for families with excessively crying, sleepless and demanding babies):
www.cry-sis.org.uk

Depression Alliance (information and support services for those suffering from depression):
www.depressionalliance.org

Counselling

British Association for Counselling and Psychotherapy:
www.bacp.co.uk

British Infertility Counselling Association:
www.bica.net

Relate (relationship counselling and advice):
www.relate.org.uk

Adoption and fostering

Adoption UK (supports adopters and prospective adopters):
www.adoptionuk.org

British Association for Adoption and Fostering:
www.baaf.org.uk

The Fostering Network:
www.fostering.net

OASIS (Overseas Adoption Support and Information Service):
www.adoptionoverseas.org

Ireland

Breastfeeding Support Network:
www.breastfeeding.ie

Irish Multiple Births Association (supports parents of multiples):
www.imba.ie

The Miscarriage Association of Ireland:
www.miscarriage.ie

Australia

Australian Multiple Birth Association (support and information to multiple-birth families):
www.amba.org.au

Childbirth Australia (aims to give women a stronger voice in childbirth issues):
http://childbirth.org.au

Donor Conception Support Group of Australia:
www.dcsg.org.au

SANDS Australian (offers miscarriage, stillbirth and neonatal-death support):
www.sands.org.au

Solo Mums by Choice Australia (support for women who have chosen to become a sole parent):
www.smcaustralia.org

Stillbirth Foundation (works to reduce the incidence of stillbirth):
www.stillbirthfoundation.org.au

New Zealand

La Leche League (breastfeeding support):
www.lalecheleague.org.nz

Miscarriage Support:
www.miscarriagesupport.org.nz

New Zealand Multiple Birth Association:
www.multiples.org.nz

SANDS New Zealand (offers support to parents and families who have experienced the death of a baby):
www.sands.org.nz

Trauma and Birth Stress (information and support after birth trauma):
www.tabs.org.nz

Twin Loss NZ (group for those who have lost one or more of multiples):
www.twinloss.org.nz

South Africa

South African Society of Obstetricians and Gynaecologists:
www.sasog.co.za

The South African Multiple Birth Association:
www.samultiplebirth.co.za

US

American Pregnancy Association (advice and information about pregnancy):
www.americanpregnancy.org

Babyloss (support for anyone affected by the loss of a baby):
www.babyloss.com

The National Organisation of Mothers of Twins Clubs (support group for parents of twins and higher order multiples):
www.nomotc.org

La Leche League (breastfeeding support):
www.llli.org

Single Mothers by Choice (group for women who have chosen to be a sole parent):
http://singlemothersbychoice.com

The Triplet Connection (support for multiple-birth families):
www.tripletconnection.org

Index